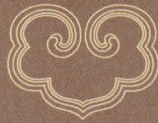

中医养生学具有悠久的历史、
独特的理论知识、丰富多彩的方法、
卓有成效的实践经验、鲜明的东方色彩
和浓郁的民族风格，是中华民族的一大
创造，是中国传统文化中的瑰宝，
也是中医学宝库中的一颗璀璨明珠。

With a long history, unique theoretical knowledge, colorful methods, fruitful practical experience, bright oriental color and rich national style, TCM health preservation is a great creation of the Chinese nation, a treasure in Chinese traditional culture and a bright pearl in the treasure house of TCM.

中 医
智 慧 与 健 康 丛书

TCM

Wisdom and Health

Series

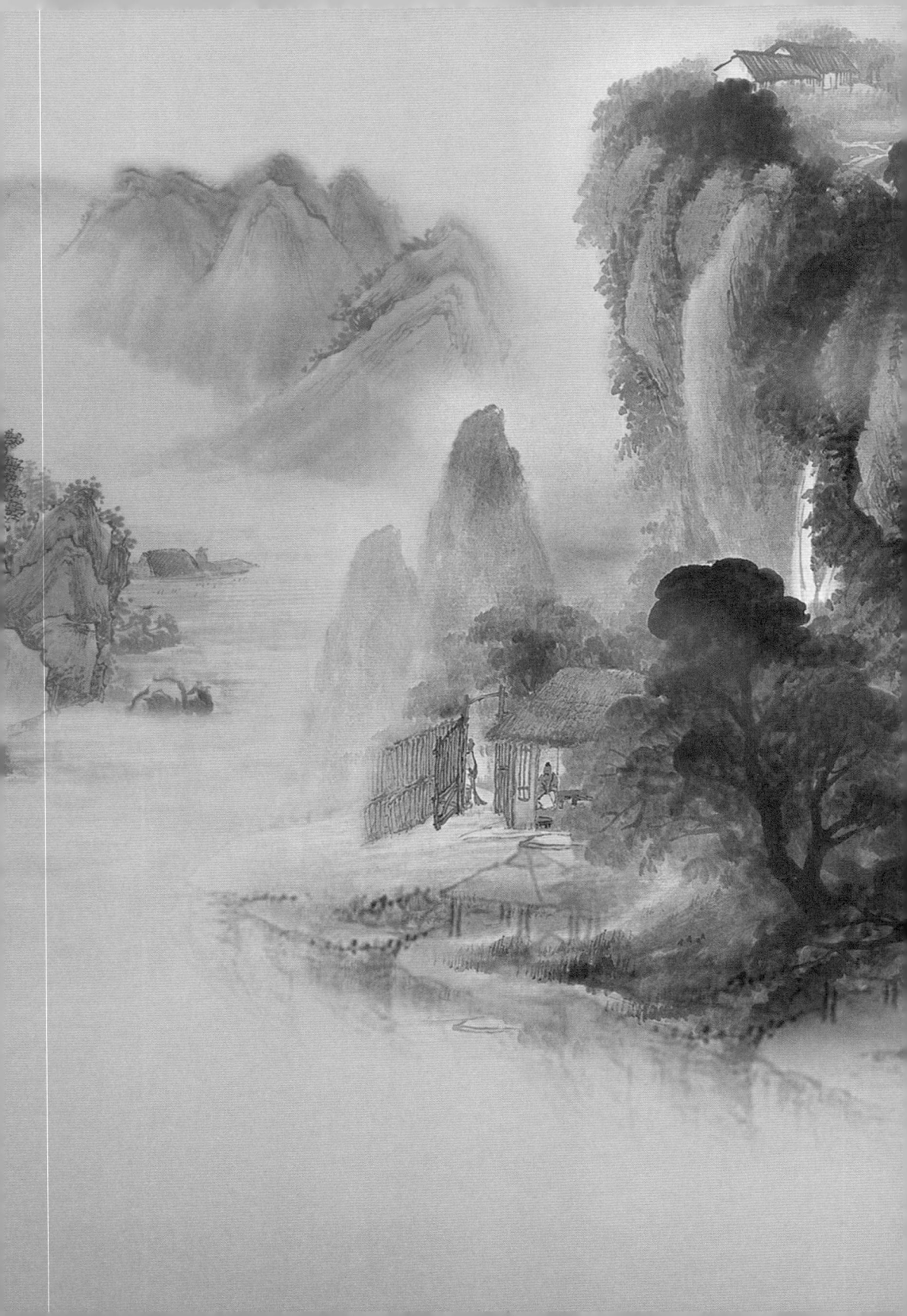

中医养生

（汉英对照）

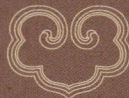

TCM Health Preservation

主　编　王笑频　尹　璐　冯　博

副主编　李　军　李　莉　冯　玲

编　委　（按姓氏笔画排序）

　　　　习亚炜　王秋虹　王笑频　尹　璐　冯　玲

　　　　冯　博　刘　瑞　刘　超　李　军　李　莉

　　　　罗富锟　胡　骏　钱晶晶　高　扬　高学成

Chief Editors

Wang Xiaopin　Yin Lu　Feng Bo

Associate Editors

Li Jun　Li Li　Feng Ling

Editorial Board

(Listed in order of surname stroke)

Xi Yawei	Wang Qiuhong	Wang Xiaopin	Yin Lu	Feng Ling
Feng Bo	Liu Rui	Liu Chao	Li Jun	Li Li
Luo Fukun	Hu Jun	Qian Jingjing	Gao Yang	Gao Xuecheng

人民卫生出版社
PMPH　PEOPLE'S MEDICAL PUBLISHING HOUSE

图书在版编目（CIP）数据

中医养生：汉英对照 / 王笑频，尹璐，冯博主编 .
北京：人民卫生出版社，2025. 5. --（中医智慧与健康
丛书）. -- ISBN 978-7-117-37456-9

Ⅰ. R212

中国国家版本馆 CIP 数据核字第 202559CE91 号

人卫智网	www.ipmph.com	医学教育、学术、考试、健康，购书智慧智能综合服务平台
人卫官网	www.pmph.com	人卫官方资讯发布平台

中医养生（汉英对照）
Zhongyi Yangsheng（Han-Ying Duizhao）

主　　编：王笑频　尹　璐　冯　博
出版发行：人民卫生出版社（中继线 010-59780011）
地　　址：北京市朝阳区潘家园南里 19 号
邮　　编：100021
E - mail：pmph @ pmph.com
购书热线：010-59787592　010-59787584　010-65264830
印　　刷：北京华联印刷有限公司
经　　销：新华书店
开　　本：710×1000　1/16　印张：17
字　　数：333 千字
版　　次：2025 年 5 月第 1 版
印　　次：2025 年 6 月第 1 次印刷
标准书号：ISBN 978-7-117-37456-9
定　　价：128.00 元
打击盗版举报电话：010-59787491　E-mail：WQ @ pmph.com
质量问题联系电话：010-59787234　E-mail：zhiliang @ pmph.com
数字融合服务电话：4001118166　E-mail：zengzhi @ pmph.com

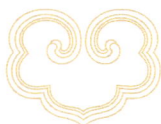

序

  中医药蕴含着数千年来中华民族治病疗疾、养生保健的智慧，护佑着中华儿女生生不息，是中华民族的伟大创造与中国古代科学的瑰宝。"中医智慧与健康丛书"正是为了系统总结中医药千年来的实践经验与临床智慧、科学普及中医药知识所编撰。

  本丛书由中国中医科学院广安门医院牵头撰写，依托国家中医药管理局国际合作司中医药国际合作专项，通过《中医史话》《中华本草》《中医诊疗》《中医养生》四个分册，全方位展示了中医药历史传承、特色优势和优秀成果，旨在向国内外读者普及中医药文化，促进中医药文化的国际传播，做好文明互鉴。丛书精心选取内容，语言通俗易懂，图文并茂，采用中英双语对照的形式，以方便国内外读者阅读。

  我们真诚地希望通过本丛书，广大读者朋友能够更好地了解中医、用上中医、爱上中医，成为中医的"粉丝"。

"中医智慧与健康丛书"编委会
2023 年 6 月

TCM Wisdom
and
Health Series

Foreword

Traditional Chinese medicine (TCM) contains the wisdom of the Chinese nation in treating diseases and maintaining health for thousands of years, and protects the endless survival of the Chinese people. It is the great creation of the Chinese nation and the treasure of ancient Chinese science. **The TCM Wisdom and Health Series** is compiled to systematically summarize the practical experience and clinical wisdom of TCM and popularize the knowledge of TCM.

This series is compiled under the leadership of Guang'anmen Hospital of China Academy of Chinese Medical Sciences (CACMS). Relying on the Special International Cooperation Project of TCM of Department of International Cooperation of National Administration of Traditional Chinese Medicine, the series shows the historical inheritance, characteristic advantages and outstanding achievements of TCM in an all-round way ranging from history, materia medica, diagnosis and treatment of TCM to health cultivation, aiming to popularize Chinese medical culture to readers at home and abroad, promote the international communication of Chinese medical culture as well as mutual learning among civilizations. The series carefully selects content, uses language easy to understand, illustrates texts with pictures, and adopts the bilingual form of both Chinese and English to facilitate readers at home and abroad.

We sincerely hope by reading this series readers can better understand TCM, use TCM, fall in love with TCM, and become the "fans" of TCM.

Editorial Board of **TCM Wisdom and Health Series**
June 2023

前言

中医养生学是以中国古代天文、地理、文化、历史、哲学为深厚底蕴，以中医理论为坚实基础，集各地、各民族的养生智慧于一体，融汇道家、儒家、佛家及历代养生家、医学家和广大劳动人民长期的防病保健的养生体验和实践成果，逐步形成的博大精深的理论体系。中医养生学具有悠久的历史、独特的理论知识、丰富多彩的方法、卓有成效的实践经验、鲜明的东方色彩和浓郁的民族风格，是中华民族的一大创造，是中国传统文化中的瑰宝，也是中医学宝库中的一颗璀璨明珠。在绵延数千年的历史长河中，中医养生学为中华民族的繁衍昌盛和健康事业做出了不可磨灭的卓越贡献。

健康与长寿历来是人类永恒的向往和追求。《北史》云："人之所宝，莫宝于生命。"生命对于每个人来说都仅有一次。人类始终在不断地努力探索健康长寿的途径和方法。养生的根本目的就是保持健康、益寿延年。养生的意义重大，不可忽视。

近年来，随着经济、科学文化的快速发展，现代社会节奏加快，加之环境污染、营养过剩，许多现代病随之而来。老年人口占总人口的比例越来越大，全球人口老龄化的趋势日益严峻，人口老龄化又向世界医学发出挑战，迫切地需要解决人们防病、治病、养生、保健的问题。对此，西医学曾做出过很大努力，但还不能满足养生保健的需要。中国中医药有几千年的历史，具有丰富的养生知识和方法。随着社会的进步和时代的发展，以及生命科学的研究进展和医疗卫生工作重心的前移，中医养生学的价值更加凸显，已成为一门充满生机与活力的中医分支学科。在当前形势下，以科学的态度和方法，传承和发展中医养生学，让中医养生智慧为更多人带来健康生活，具有重要的现实意义和社会意义。

本书以问题形式展示中医养生的核心内容，图文并茂，包括中医养生学的形成与发展、中医养生基本概念、养形、养神、食养、药养、针灸养生、其他非药物养生方法等，以期使读者全面了解中医养生。

由于编写人员的水平所限，书内难免有挂一漏万之处，欢迎各位读者批评指正。

《中医养生》编写委员会
2023 年 6 月

Preface

Health preservation of traditional Chinese medicine (TCM) is a wonderful work of Chinese traditional culture. Taking China's ancient astronomy, geography, culture, history and philosophy as its profound foundation, with its theory as solid foundation, it integrates the health-preserving wisdom of various places and nationalities, and the health-preserving experiences and research achievements of Taoism, Confucianism, Buddhism, past generations of health-preserving experts and medical scientists, as well as ordinary people to form a profound theoretical system. With a long history, unique theoretical knowledge, colorful methods, fruitful practical experience, bright oriental color and rich national style, TCM health preservation is a great creation of the Chinese nation, a treasure in Chinese traditional culture and a bright pearl in the treasure house of TCM. In the long history of thousands of years, TCM health preservation has made indelible and outstanding contributions to the prosperity and health of the Chinese nation.

Health and longevity have always been the eternal yearning and pursuit of mankind. *Northern History* goes: "The treasure of a man is the treasure of life." Life is only once for everyone. Human beings are constantly trying to explore ways and means to live a long and healthy life. The fundamental purpose of preserving health is to keep healthy and live longer. Keeping in good health is of great significance and cannot be ignored.

In recent years, with the rapid development of economy, science and culture, the fast pace of modern society, coupled with environmental pollution, excessive nutrition, many modern diseases have followed. The proportion of the elderly population in the total population is increasing, and the trend of global population aging is increasing day by day. The aging society challenges the world's medicine, and it is urgent to solve the problems of disease prevention, treatment, health preservation and health care for all people. In this regard, modern medicine has made great efforts, but it still can not meet the needs of health care. TCM in China has a history of thousands of years, and is rich in knowledge and methods of health preservation. With the progress of the society and the development of the times, as well as the research progress of life sciences and the shift of the focus of medical and health work, the value of TCM health preservation has become more prominent, and it has become a branch of TCM full of vitality and vigor. Especially in the new situation, TCM health preservation has more important practical and social significance. We should inherit, study and develop the knowledge of TCM health preservation with a scientific attitude and method, so as to carry forward the health preservation of TCM, enabling the wisdom of TCM health preservation to bring a healthy lifestyle to more people.

This book displays the core content of TCM health preservation in the form of questions, and shows the brief history of TCM health preservation, the foundamentals of TCM health preservation, cultivating the body, cultivating the spirit, diatetic health preservation, medications for health preservation, acupuncture and moxibustion for health preservatioin, and other non-medication therapy for health preservation. We hope readers can get a comprehensive understanding of TCM health preservation from this book.

Due to the limited skills of our writers, it is inevitable that there will be mistakes in the book. Readers are welcome to criticize and correct them.

Editorial Board of
TCM Health Preservation
June 2023

目 录

Contents

目　录

Contents

Contents

中医养生

（汉英对照）

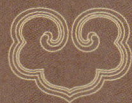

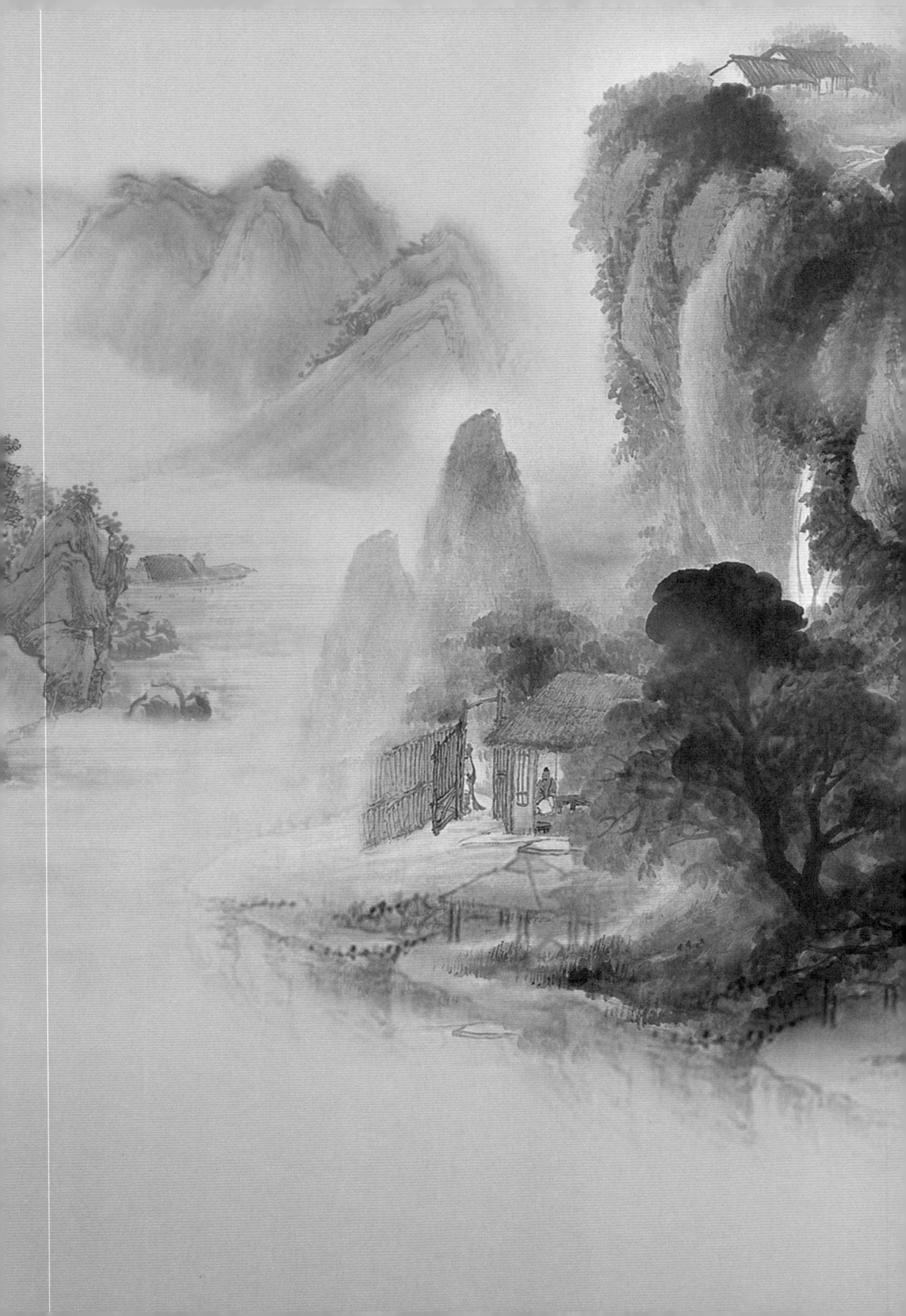

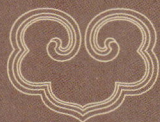

第一章

中医养生学的形成与发展

中医养生学起源于何时？

中医养生学的起源，可追溯到春秋以前。在原始社会里，生产力极为低下，远古人类过着茹毛饮血的生活，但作为一种本能需要，已促使人类依靠自己的主观能动性去认识自然、适应自然，在劳动实践中不断探索、不断实践，探求人类自身发展以至种族生存和延续的各种手段和方法，达到却病延年的目的。在已出土的殷商时期的甲骨文中已有"沐""浴"等体现当时人们卫生活动的文字，表明中国早在公元前十四世纪就已有了养生防病的措施。到原始社会末期，人们已经知道用宣导、运动的方法来防病治病，如《吕氏春秋·古乐》记载："昔陶唐氏之始，阴多滞伏而湛积，水道壅塞，不行其原，民气郁阏而滞著，筋骨瑟缩不达，故作为舞以宣导之。"所谓"舞"，就是活动关节，是使气血通畅的一种导引术雏形。《神仙传》等书还记载，远古彭祖因养生之道，活了八百岁。从今天的观点来看，人活八百岁不太可能，但至少说明早在远古时期，养生之道就已为人们所重视。岐伯与黄帝的一段对话提到"上古之人，其知道者……度百岁乃去"（《素问·上古天真论》），其中的"道"，就是今天所说的养生方法。但是，在春秋以前，完整的医学体系尚未形成，治疗手段也很原始，故春秋以前的养生学尚处于萌芽时期。这一时期的养生特点是顺应自然，以饮食调养和宣导为主。

道家思想如何主导中医养生学的形成？

道家泛指以先秦老子、庄子学说为中心的哲学流派。道家学说的创始人，一般认为是老子。老子，姓李，名耳，生活于春秋时代，代表作是《道德经》，其学术思想基本属于自然主义的哲学。战国时期的庄周，继承和发扬了老子的思想，这一时期的道家思想称为"老庄哲学"。"养生"一词，最早见于《庄子·内篇·养生主》，专论养生；《庄子·外篇·刻意》云："吹呴呼吸，吐故纳新，熊经鸟申，为寿而已矣。"均是其养生思想的阐述。道家思想对中医养生学的形

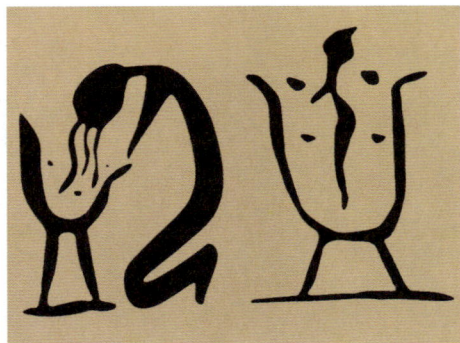

甲骨文中的"沐"（左图）、"浴"（右图）

成与发展的影响是巨大的。道家所主张的"道"，是指天地万物的本质及其自然循环的规律。自然界的万事万物都处于运动变化之中，"道"即是其基本法则。《道德经》云"人法地，地法天，天法道，道法自然"，就是关于"道"的具体阐述。所以，人的生命活动应当符合自然规律，方能长寿，这是道家思想的根本观念。道家思想中，清静无为、返璞归真、顺应自然、贵柔及动形达郁等主张对中医养生学有很大的影响。道家思想对中医养生学的影响主要体现在以下几个方面：一是提出了精、气、神等基本概念；二是创立了静态养生法；三是崇尚自然，创立了顺乎自然的气功养生法，兼养形神；四是主张贵"柔"；五是从哲学上阐述了养生的意义和原则。

探讨养生史，学习养生术，道家的作用是不能忽视的，但须注意道家早期老庄养生法中含有消极顺应自然的思想，在具体研究和实践中应注意匡正。

儒家思想如何促进中医养生理论形成？

以孔孟为代表的儒家学派，一直是中国古代思想史上的中坚学派，儒学也成为封建社会统治数千年的"官学"，对中国的政治和文化产生了深远的影响。其对医学也产生了重大的影响，医学史上就有"医儒不分"的说法。由于儒家主张以"中庸"为修身养性之法，并且儒家的鼻祖孔子又是养生的主张者和力行者，因此儒家的养生方法丰富了中医养生学的内容，促进了中医养生理论的形成。

儒家对中医养生学影响最深莫过于"中和观"。《中庸》是专门论述中和观的著作。《史记·孔子世家》载："子思作《中庸》。"子思即孔子的孙子，又名孔伋，孔子的中和思想就是由他保留记录下来的。所谓"中庸"，是儒家讲人性修养的一种境界——"和而不流""中立不倚"，既毋太过，也毋不及。《中庸》曰："喜怒哀乐之未发，谓之中；发而皆中节，谓之和。中和者，天下之大本也。和也者，天下之达道也。致中和，天地位焉，万物育焉。"就是说，只要人的修养达到中和的境界，就会产生"天地位焉，万物育焉"的效果。《黄帝内经》在讨论上古之人长寿的原因时指出"上古之人，其知道者，法于阴阳，和于术数"，这个"和"字，很可能是儒家中和观运用于养生学最早的记载，即通过"术数"达到"和"的境界，使阴不虚，阳不亢，而"度百岁乃去"，后世医家也多次在著作中提到"和"的养生理论，可见其影响之深。

儒家思想丰富了中医养生学的内容，促进了中医养生理论的形成，其主要学术思想和观念有三点。一是强调精神调摄。孔子非常注重精神养生，提倡修身养性和道德修养。孟子更是重视"养心"，"苟得其养，无物不长；苟失其养，无物不消"（《孟子·告子上》），其养心的具体方法是"养心莫善于寡欲。其为人也寡欲，虽有不存焉者，寡矣"（《孟子·尽心下》）。后世儒家代表董仲舒、程颐、朱熹及医家孙思邈等人进一步将其思想发挥，与养生方法相联系，形成了具有儒家特色的养生流派。孔子还提出"三戒"思想，曰"君子有三戒：少之时，血气未定，戒之在色；及其壮也，血气方刚，戒之在斗；及其老也，血气既衰，戒之在得"（《论语·季氏》）。二是注重身体养护。这是儒家"中和观"思想的具体体现。起居有常、劳逸适度、饮食有节等是护养身体的基本原则，在儒家"中和观"养生思想的影响下，形成了丰富的养生理论、原则和方法。如宋代严用和《济生方》云："善摄生者，谨于和调，一饮一食，使入于胃中，随消随化，则无滞留之患；若禀受怯弱，饥饱失时，或过餐五味，鱼腥乳酪，强食生冷果菜，停蓄胃脘，遂成宿滞。"就是在儒家思想影响下形成的饮食中和观。此外，还有《养性延命录》中"能中和者必久寿"，《医述》中"人生如天地，和煦则春，惨郁则秋"等论述。三是孔子在饮食养生方面有独到见解。孔子对于饮食卫生提出"食不厌精，脍不厌细，食饐而餲，鱼馁而肉败，不食。色恶，不食；失饪，不食；不时，不食"（《论语·乡党》）。后世的饮食养生观有许多是从孔子饮食养生方面的创见中发展起来的，如"食精则能养人，脍粗则能害人"（《退庵随笔》），"饮食之宜，当候已饥而进食，食不厌细嚼。仍候焦渴而引饮，饮不厌细呷"（《饮食以宜》）。

儒家养生思想，特别是儒家"中和观"，为历代医家所遵循，对后世养生学的发展有很大的影响，时至今日仍有其实用价值。

《黄帝内经》对中医养生学有什么影响？

在《黄帝内经》以前，养生学处于实践阶段，尚无系统的养生理论。《黄帝内经》一书，全面汲取了秦汉以前的养生学成就，对于中医养生学的有关理论、方法和原则进行了比较全面而系统的论述。因此，《黄帝内经》的成书是中医养生史上的里程碑，它为中医养生学的形成奠定了坚实的理论基础。

《黄帝内经》对中医养生学的贡献主要体现在以下方面：

第一，强调精、气、神人身三宝。《黄帝内经》认为精是构成人体的基本物质，"人始生，先成精，精成而脑髓生"（《灵枢·经脉》）。精又是人体生命活动的原始动力，是身体强壮、不老延年的本源，"夫精者身之本也"（《素问·金匮真言论》）。气，指精微物质，又指脏腑活动的能力。人的生命结束就是"五脏皆虚，神气皆去，形骸独居而终矣"（《灵枢·天年》）。神为生命活动现象的总称，是精神、意识、知觉、运动等一切生命活动的集中表现。"得神者昌，失神者亡"(《素问·移精变气论》)。可见，精、气、神是人体至贵三宝，后世养生家多注重养精、益气、治神。

第二，确立了"天人相应"的养生原则。《黄帝内经》把人和自然界看成一个整体，即天有所变，人有所应。其认为养生的要旨是"顺四时而适寒暑，和喜怒而安居处，节阴阳而调刚柔"(《灵枢·本神》)，并提出了著名的"春夏养阳，秋冬养阴"的四时顺养原则，《素问·上古天真论》又明确指出"虚邪贼风，避之有时"，开辟了防病治病先河。

第三，阐述了生命规律。《黄帝内经》对人体生、长、壮、老、已的生命规律有精妙的观察和科学的概括。《灵枢·天年》把人的生长发育分为十个阶段，每个阶段为十年。《素问·阴阳应象大论》也基本采用了十年为期的划分法。而《素问·上古天真论》则以女七、男八为周期。这些是中国医学史上最早的关于人体生长、发育、衰老的周期划分，为以后中医养生学研究生命规律及老年病学防老抗衰提供了借鉴。

第四，创立了经络学说，为气功、导引、按摩等非药物养生疗法奠定理论基础。长沙马王堆出土的帛书《足臂十一脉灸经》《阴阳十一脉灸经》，虽然成书早于《黄帝内经》，但内容简单，未形成系统的经络学说。《黄帝内经》则形成了系统完整的经络学说，它分为十二正经、奇经八脉等内容，并指出经络的作用是"行血气而营阴阳，濡筋骨，利关节"(《灵枢·本脏》)。

第五，总结、保留了战国以前许多行之有效的养生方法和原则。如"恬惔虚无，真气从之，精神内守"就是对道家精神养生方法的总结。此外，还提出食养与食疗、动静结合、形体锻炼等行之有效的养生原则和方法。

《黄帝内经》对中医养生学的贡献是巨大的，它牢固奠定了中医养生学的理论基础。此后，尽管中医养生学在理论上有所提高，在方法上有所创新，但始终是以《黄帝内经》为理论指导。

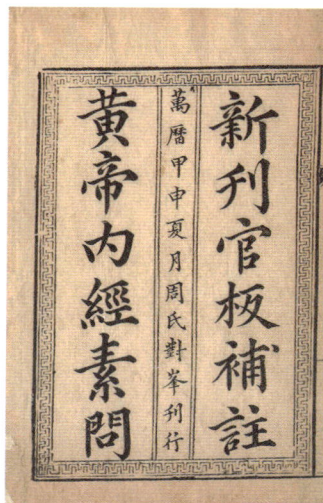

新刊官板補註
萬曆甲申夏月周氏對峰刊行
黄帝内經素問

《黄帝内经素问》

吐纳导引术如何促进中医养生学的发展？

《黄帝内经》总结了萌发、流传的吐纳导引术，肯定了上古之人"尽终其天年，度百岁乃去"的重要措施是"和于术数"。吐纳导引术就是术数之一，吐纳导引术的却病机理是"真气从之，精神内守"，导引术的主要方法是调神（心）、调气（息）和调身，即"呼吸精气，独立守神，肌肉若一"（《素问·上古天真论》）。

战国时期，由于道教的兴起，这一时期的吐纳导引术，乃至其后的气功都有一个鲜明的特点，就是糅合了道家"清静无为"思想。

汉代、三国的导引术秉承战国、秦代，但在理论和方法上有所创新。仲景对导引吐纳也十分重视，主张用动形养生的方法防病治病，如"四肢才觉重滞，即导引吐纳……勿令九窍闭塞"（《金匮要略》）。东汉时期的王充、华佗等对《黄帝内经》的养生学说作了某些补充和发挥，推动了吐纳导引术的发展。王充在《论衡》中专门探讨有关健康和寿命的问题，其中论及生死寿夭、延年之道者近二十篇，如《论衡·气寿》云："夫禀气渥则体强，体强则其命长；气薄则其体弱，体弱则命短。"明确提出了先天禀赋强者寿长，先天禀赋弱者寿短的观点。并在《自纪》中载"养气自守，适时则酒。闭明塞聪，爱精自保。适辅服药引导，庶冀性命可延，斯须不老"，记录了他本人"养气自守""服药引导"的一些方法。汉末史学家荀悦《申鉴·俗嫌》中有"邻脐二寸谓之关，道家常致气于关，是为要求"，表明当时已注意到气功与经络穴位的关系，并已出现气贯关元、意守关元等功法。华佗是与张仲景同时期的一位著名的医家、养生家，他继承《吕氏春秋》提出的"流水不腐，户枢不蠹"的思想，从理论上进一步阐述了动形养生的道理。《三国志·华佗传》载："人体欲得劳动，但不当使极尔，动摇则谷气得消，血脉流通，病不得生，譬犹户枢不朽是也。"他还继承《庄子》"吐故纳新，熊经鸟申"的思想，创立了动形养生的五禽戏。五禽戏是仿效虎、鹿、熊、猿、鸟五种动物的动作锻炼身体，虎戏勇猛力大，威武刚健，常练可使四肢粗壮，增强气力；鹿戏动作舒展，姿态动静相兼，常练可使腰腿灵活，神态自然，体形健美；熊戏步履沉稳，力撼山岳，常练可增强抵抗能力和耐久性；猿戏机灵敏捷，跳跃自如，喜搓颜面，常练可使头脑清醒，反应灵敏，动作轻灵；鸟戏模仿空中飞鸟，悠然自得，上下翻飞，常练使人体态轻盈。五禽戏经长期的流传和发展，既可防病治病，又可增强身体素质，将导引术向前推进了一步。

魏晋南北朝时期，导引术在理论、内容和方法上又有了进一步的发展。嵇康的《养生论》涉及大量导引的内容，阐述了"导养得理，以尽性命"的道理。

葛洪在《抱朴子》一书中对气功有许多精辟的论述，指出气功的作用是"内以养身，外以祛邪"，探讨了导引的机理是"宣动营卫"，他还提倡导引术应动静结合，不拘形式，"或屈伸，或俯仰，或行卧，或倚立，或踯躅，或徐步，或吟，或息，皆导引也"，对后世导引术形式多样化产生了一定影响。晋代还有一位叫许逊的道士，其所著《净明宗教录》中也载有一些导引方法，尤其是"气功若成，筋骨和柔，百关通畅"中的"气功"二字，很可能是现存文献中"气功"二字最早的记载。

至隋唐时期，导引术得到了朝廷的正式承认，确定作为一种养生及医疗手段。由于朝廷的重视及长期实践丰富的积累，隋唐时代导引术的发展达到高峰。隋朝太医博士巢元方《诸病源候论》所论述的1729种病候中，其他疗法、方法或简述，或未述，唯有"补养宣导"的方法，则几乎在每种疾病中都附有内容具体、形象生动、具有实效的说明。唐代大医孙思邈，也是一位十分讲究导引的养生家。在《备急千金要方》和《摄养枕中方》中都载录了大量涉及导引和行气的内容。此外，在《备急千金要方》中还记录了佛家功的一些内容，表明这一时期，吐纳导引术已出现了多流派并存的局面。

总之，在远古时代萌芽的吐纳导引术，经过春秋战国、秦汉、魏晋南北朝的不断积累和发展，到隋唐时代已成为中医养生学的重要组成部分，并得以不断普及和提高。

中医养生流派有哪些？

随着《黄帝内经》的成书，中医养生学在战国时期迎来了其发展史上的第一个高峰，道家、儒家思想也渗入到养生学中，与养生理论融合，初步形成了不同风格的养生观点和方法。为了研究和继承方便，采用医学史上通常划分流派的方法将中医养生流派划分为道家养生派、佛家养生派、儒家养生派、医家养生派。然而各流派之间无严格界限，特别在唐代儒、佛、道存在着"三教合一"的趋势下，许多养生家及养生著作也是兼收并蓄的。

道家养生派的思想特点是什么？

从秦朝开始，道家思想首先得到重视。许多信奉老庄思想的学者和方士，大力提倡导引、吐纳等养生方法，如张良、李少君、东方朔等。嵇康在《养生论》中重申了老庄学派的养生理论和方法。葛洪《抱朴子》广泛论述了道家的各种养生理论和方法，使正统的道家养生术得以系统发展。如果把老子、庄子称为道家养生派的奠基人，葛洪则是其当然的代表人物了。

佛家养生派的思想特点是什么？

佛教产生于印度，经由中亚传入中国新疆，西汉末年传入内地（传入年代参考翦伯赞主编《中国史纲要》）。佛教传入中国后，最早是与黄老学说并列的，民间流传有"老子入夷为浮屠"之说，因此尽管佛家养生法随着佛教的传入而有所流传，但早期多依附于道家养生法中，无大发展。至隋唐时期，才开始异军突起，并作为养生流派分化而独立。孙思邈《备急千金要方》中收入了天竺国按摩法。此外，尚有达摩易筋经、天台宗六妙法门、西藏密宗金刚拳等养生方法，都是属于佛家养生术的范畴。

儒家养生派的思想特点是什么？

儒家养生的宗旨是中和观和修身养性，在战国时期，儒家只是作为"九流十家"中的一个流派存在，尚处于萌芽阶段。到汉代，汉武帝时期董仲舒提出"独尊儒术"，汉建元五年（公元前136年）设置五经博士，把儒学抬高为官学，随着儒学地位的上升，儒家养生派也开始逐渐分化为一个独立流派。首先是董仲舒将养生和中庸思想相结合，强调养气与中和。成书于西汉的《淮南子》，尽管倾向于"以道绌儒"，但书中对儒家的许多合理部分作了尽情发挥，发展了儒家的修身养性理论。而后荀悦把儒家的养性学说与气、形、神等相结合，并从理论上作了阐述，使儒家的养性学说与人体生理病理变化联系更为紧密，更便于推广。到隋唐时期，儒家养生派在官场、文人中已经很盛行了。唐代著名医家、养生家孙思邈是一个儒、释、道兼而融之的人物，其所著《备急千金要方》专列养生一卷，名之曰"养性"。至宋代，经过程颐、朱熹、陆九渊、王守仁等人的补充、发挥，儒家养生学更加盛行。总之，儒家养生派是从西汉以后，历代儒生把孔孟学说中的道德修养、道德意识及中和观等思想与中医养生方法联系在一起而逐渐形成的，它与中医养生学既有必然联系，又具有自己的特色。

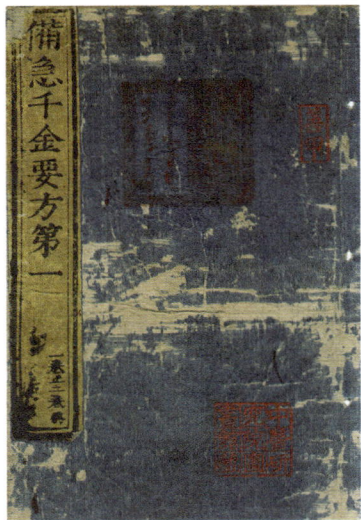

《备急千金要方》
中国中医科学院藏

医家养生派思想特点是什么？

医家养生派是指以药物、饮食为主要手段的养生流派。在医家养生派中，又有许多细的分支，以饮食调养为主者称为食养派，以药物调补为主者称为药养派，在药养派中，因用药习惯的不同又分为理脾、补肾、养阴、壮阳诸家。

宋金元、明清时期养生保健学如何充实和发展？

宋金元时期是中国封建社会后期，在思想上倡导熔道、佛、儒三教于一炉的所谓"理学"，又出现"新学"哲学流派，它们既有争论，又相互渗透，互相吸收和发扬，对医疗保健有一定影响。宋代以后，养生保健的重点开始转移，到明清时期，基本形成了独具特色的老年养生学体系。与此同时，食物养生不断地深化和普及，食养的理论、品谱、方法更加完善。由于金元时期医学流派的兴起，对中医养生学，尤其是医家养生流派产生了很大的影响。宋金元至明清时期是中医养生学发展的黄金时期，是中国古代历史上养生学发展速度最快的时期，出现了很多著名养生家。这一时期养生学特点如下。

第一，养生保健方法日臻完备。北宋宫廷编著的方剂专书《太平圣惠方》，不仅是一部具有理、法、方、药完整体系的医书，且载有许多摄生保健的内容。北宋末年，政府组织编写了《圣济总录》，共 200 卷，200 余万字，包括内、外、妇、儿、五官、针灸及养生、杂治等 66 门，内容十分丰富，书中对养生保健的一些方法做了相当详尽的介绍。

第二，老年养生保健进一步充实和发展。金元时期，学术争鸣，对老年人的养生理论和方法有了更趋完善的认识，主要表现在以下几个方面：强调精神调摄，主张饮食调养，提倡顺时奉养，重视起居护养，注意药物扶持。

第三，纠正了药物养生的不良倾向。这一时期服饵金石的不良倾向逐渐得到纠正，使药物养生走上了正轨。

第四，食养方法的丰富和普及。由于实践经验的不断积累，食养食疗在理论和方法上均有了新的发展，取得了显著的成就。

第五，金元四大家对养生学产生了较大影响。他们不仅是临床家、理论家，也是养生家，对养生学理论的创新和发展起了很大的作用。其中刘完素主张养生重在养气，张子和提倡祛邪扶正，李东垣注重调理脾胃，朱丹溪强调阴气保养。

现当代养生学如何复兴发展？

中华人民共和国成立后，中医养生事业受到政府重视，相应的机构开始建立，养生的书籍、论文日益增多，养生术逐渐普及。到 20 世纪 50 年代中期，随着经济文化建设逐渐走上正轨，中医养生事业开始复苏，由于这一时期受财力、物力限制，中医药工作的重点是治疗那些危害劳动人民身体健康的常见病、多发病。故花钱少、普及快的气功养生率先兴起，1957 年 7 月上海市气功疗养所成立，标志着中国气功养生走上了一个新台阶。该养生所成立后，开展了一些引人注目的气功养生项目，并对气功与经络的关系，以及对经络的探测与证实问题进行了探讨。这一时期出版了大量的中医书籍，兴起了西学中热并促进了中医养生研究的发展。

20 世纪 70 年代末期，党和国家的工作重点转移到以经济建设为中心，将改革开放作为基本国策，成为中国社会主义建设的基本思想，党和政府尊重科学、重视科学，科学的春天到来了，中医养生学的春天也到来了。加上这一时期国际老年医学发展很快，社会老龄化趋势明显，给中医养生学带来动力和机遇。1980 年 6 月，中国中医研究院西苑医院成立了岳美中学术经验研究室，开始从事中医老年医学和抗衰老医药研究，曾先后发表了《补益类长寿植物药概述》《抗衰老动物药概述》等论文，后者还被译为日文在日本发表。80 年代以来，一方面，对古代养生方面的珍本、善本进行整理出版；另一方面，今人的研究专著也不断问世，大大推动了这一时期中医养生学的发展。1988 年 4 月，在山东青岛召开了中国首届康复疗养养生学术研讨会，全国康复、疗养、养生专家薛效勤、王凤岐、王育学、孙光荣等 120 余人云集一堂，交流了养生学研究成果。

近年来，随着医学模式的转变，医学科学研究的重点已开始从临床逐渐转向预防医学和康复医学，传统的养生保健得到更加迅速的发展，出现了蓬勃向上的局面，概括起来，主要有以下几个方面：一是预防保健取得显著成就；二是建立养生保健的科研机构；三是理论研究不断取得进展；四是开展社会性保健教育；五是在养生学教育上有所创树；六是积极开展学术交流活动。中医养生学的不断发展，将会为中国及世界人民的健康延寿做出更大的贡献。

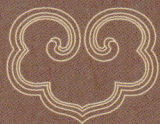

第二章

中医养生学基本概念

第一节
天 年

什么是自然寿命？

自然寿命的含义是：在没有任何意外使生命缩短的情况下，从第一次呼吸到最后一次呼吸的间期。在中国古代文献中，常将自然寿命称为"天年"。

人类应享的自然寿命是多少？

《素问·上古天真论》指出"尽终其天年，度百岁乃去"；《灵枢·天年》亦云"人之寿百岁而死"；汉代也有"强弱天寿，以百为数"之说。《老子》则提出"人生大期，以百二十为限"；《尚书·洪范》载"一曰寿，百二十岁也"。可见中国古代医家、学者认为人类"天年"的限度为 100~120 岁。

衰老的分界线是什么？

每个人都要经历出生、发育、成长、衰老、死亡这样一个生命历程，衰老是生命发展过程的一个阶段，那么这个阶段是从什么时候算起呢？

《灵枢·天年》记载："人生十岁，五脏始定，血气以通，其气在下，故好走……四十岁，五脏六腑、十二经脉，皆大盛以平定，腠理始疏，荣华颓落，发颇斑白，平盛不摇，故好坐；五十岁，肝气始衰，肝叶始薄，胆汁始减，目始不明；六十岁，心气始衰，苦忧悲，血气懈堕，故好卧；七十岁，脾气虚，皮肤枯；八十岁，肺气衰，魄离，故言善误；九十岁，肾气焦，四脏经脉空虚；百岁，五脏皆虚……"将人体生命历程以十岁为单位来划分，认为到四十岁，虽然机体发育处于鼎盛时期，但也开始出现衰老征象。《素问·上古天真论》曰："女子七岁，肾气盛，齿更发长；二七而天癸至，任脉通，太冲脉盛，月事以时下，故有子；三七，肾气平均，故真牙生而长极；四七，筋骨坚，发长极，身体盛壮；五七，阳明脉衰，面始焦，发始堕；六七，三阳脉衰于上，面皆焦，发始白；七七，任脉虚，太冲脉衰少，天癸竭，地道不通，故形坏而无子也。丈夫八岁，肾气实，发长齿更；二八，肾气盛，天癸至，精气溢泻，阴阳和，故能有子；三八，肾气平均，筋骨劲强，故真牙生而长极；四八，筋骨隆盛，肌肉满壮；五八，肾气衰，发堕齿槁；六八，阳气衰竭于上，面焦，发鬓颁白；七八，肝气衰，筋不能动；八八，天癸竭，精少，肾脏衰，形体皆极，则齿发去。"认为男女是有各自不同的生长发育规律的。女子从"五七"三十五岁，男子从"五八"四十岁开始由盛转衰。很明显，女子的成长周期是七年，男子是八年。不仅如此，从生命由盛到衰的时间来看，女子经历的是"七七"四十九年，男子则为"八八"六十四年。而且男子比女子还整整多了一个成长周期。所以，女子不仅成熟得早，衰老得也比男子早。在中国古代文献中，有关"老"的界线还有其他说法："七十曰老""八十曰耋"（《说文解字》），"人年五十以上为老"（《灵枢》）等。概括各家观点，基本可以认为：中医学将四十岁至五十岁作为人体由盛转衰的时期。

但是，衰老的过程是逐渐发生的，且每个人开始衰老的年龄并不相同，因此，衰老的分界线很难从年龄上来截然划分。

衰老的形态特征是什么？

人届衰老之期，其外观形态上有些什么改变呢？《素问·脉要精微论》指出："夫五脏者，身之强也，头者，精明之府，头倾视深，精神将夺矣；背者，胸中之府，背曲肩随，府将坏矣；腰者，肾之府，转摇不能，肾将惫矣；膝者，筋之府，屈伸不能，行将偻附，筋将惫矣；骨者，髓之府，不能久立，行则振掉，骨将惫矣。"形象地描述了因脏腑功能减退而导致的各种衰老的体态。

《格致余论·养老论》曰："头昏目眵，肌痒溺数，鼻涕牙落，涎多寐少，足弱耳聩，健忘眩晕，肌燥面垢，发脱眼花，久坐兀睡，未风先寒，食则易饥，笑则有泪，但是老境，无不有此。"较全面地概括了人至"老境"时的各种表现。

具体来说，衰老的外观特征包括：毛发变白和脱落；皮肤松弛发皱、肌肉萎缩；出现老年斑；骨退变、齿脱落；身体结构改变等。

第二节
衰老

衰老的定义是什么？

什么是衰老？国内外学者给予了多种定义，但直到目前为止，还没有一种被公认的衰老的定义。在英文中 aging（增龄）和 senescence（老化）两个单词均用于表述衰老，通常将后者用于表示动物生命晚期功能明显衰退时出现的变化，而将 aging 一词用于功能减退的过程。还有人认为，不管是生命早期还是晚期，均用 aging 表示增龄或渐老，因此，从青春期开始发生的变化称为 aging。不过在现实生活中，这两个单词常交替使用。

中医学认为衰老的原因是什么？

《素问·上古天真论》曰："余闻上古之人春秋皆度百岁，而动作不衰；今时之人，年半百而动作皆衰者，时世异耶？人将失之耶？"这是记载黄帝向岐伯请教为什么当时之人不能像远古时代的人们那样皆度百岁，而年过半百就出现衰老。这一问题的提出，引起了历代中医学家们的兴趣，对衰老的成因从许多方面进行了探讨，大致可以归为以下几种：生活失于规律、情绪失于调节、禀赋沃薄与体质强弱、地理环境与气候条件。

生活失于规律如何导致衰老？

规律而有节制的生活，对于预防和抵御疾病的发生，获得健康长寿具有十分重要的意义。《素问·上古天真论》明确指出："法于阴阳，和于术数，食饮有节，起居有常，不妄作劳，故能形与神俱，而尽终其天年，度百岁乃去。"相反，若是长期违反规律地生活，"以酒为浆，以妄为常，醉以入房，以欲竭其精，以耗散其真，不知持满，不时御神，务快其心，逆于生乐，起居无节，故半百而衰矣。"就是说，过度饮酒，必伐气血之源；醉以入房，必损精气之本；起居无节，必动摇形气而致邪侵；图快一时，不知御神，必耗散元真。这种"以妄为常"的做法，导致"半百而衰"。

生活失于规律包括哪些方面？

第一，饮食失节。众所周知，人体的生命活动主要靠从饮食中不断摄取营养物质来维持，人体的生长发育、繁衍与长寿均与摄取营养有着密切的联系，若饮食不当，则会导致疾病发生，加速衰老。

第二，饮酒过多。中医学认为适量饮酒是可以的，但饮酒过度则会对身体造成损害。《灵枢·论勇》指出"酒者水谷之精，熟谷之液也，其气慓悍，其入于胃中则胃胀，气上逆，满于胸中，肝浮胆横。"《饮膳正要》亦说"少饮为佳，多饮伤形损寿，易人本性，其毒甚也。饮酒过度，丧生之源"。故《黄帝内经》将"以酒为浆"作为"半百而衰"的原因。

第三，劳逸失常。适度的劳动锻炼和合理的休息，是保持人体精力充沛、健康长寿的重要条件，但劳逸失常，则是影响健康、导致早衰的因素之一。故《黄帝内经》强调应"形劳而不倦"，《素问·宣明五气》明确提出了"久视伤血，久卧伤气，久坐伤肉，久立伤骨，久行伤筋"的观点，其中的"久坐、久卧"即是过逸，而"久立、久行、久视"即为过劳，两者均会损害健康。因此《养性延命录》指出"养寿之法，但莫伤之而已……不欲甚劳，不欲甚逸……"。

第四，房劳过度。适当的性生活虽是本能之举、天性之举，但恣情放纵却又是早衰之因、夭寿之由。《素问·上古天真论》指出"醉以入房，以欲竭其精，以耗散其真……故半百而衰"，说明房劳过度，会耗伤人体生命活动重要的物质基础——精。肾精亏虚，则致衰老，中医学家们建议"善者养生，必保其精"。

饮食失节包括哪些方面？

饮食失节包括过饥、过饱、偏食、饮食过冷或过热。

什么是过饥？

过饥即摄食不足，不能满足人体正常生命活动的需要，气血生化之源不足，久之可致早衰。《灵枢·五味》指出"谷不入，半日则气衰，一日则气少矣"。

什么是过饱？

过饱即饮食过量，是损害人体健康导致衰老的另一个重要因素。《素问·痹论》有"饮食自倍，肠胃乃伤"之说，就是指若进食过多，超过了肠胃的承受能力，就会损伤脾胃，使其腐熟运化水谷精微的功能减弱，损害机体健康。孙思邈《千金翼方》亦谓"夜饱，损一日之寿"，告诫人们不要饱食，尤其晚餐不宜进食过多。明代敖英在《东谷赘言》中详细地指出了饮食过饱的害处："多食之人有五患：一者大便数，二者小便数，三者扰睡眠，四者身重不堪修养，五者多患食不化。"现代医学认为，过饱会加重胃肠的负担，引起消化不良，而且过饱会使血液多集中于胃肠道，而使心、脑等重要器官缺血，致精神不振，甚至导致心脑血管病发生。长期饮食过饱，超过机体需要，就会变成脂肪贮存于体内而变肥胖，从而诱发一系列影响寿命的疾病。

偏食有哪些弊端？

对于饮食的偏嗜是致病之由、衰老之因。《素问·五脏生成》曰："多食咸，则脉凝泣而变色；多食苦，则皮槁而毛拔；多食辛，则筋急而爪枯；多食酸，则肉胝䐢而唇揭；多食甘，则骨痛而发落，此五味之所伤也。故心欲苦，肺欲辛，肝欲酸，脾欲甘，肾欲咸，此五味之所合也。"指出了偏嗜五味而致脏器偏胜偏衰所产生的一系列病变，而且《素问·至真要大论》还对五味偏胜过久所致的危害性有所认识："久而增气，物化之常也，气增而久，夭之由也。"表明五味偏胜过久可致早衰夭亡。在此基础上，还对恣食肥甘厚味所致的病变做了阐述，如"有病口甘者……名曰脾瘅……此肥美之所发也，此人必数食甘美而多肥也。肥者令人内热，甘者令人中满"（《素问·奇病论》）；"高粱之变，足生大丁"（《素问·生气通天论》）。

饮食过冷或过热对身体有什么影响？

饮食过冷或过热，均可对身体造成危害，对此，《黄帝内经》亦有论述，如"水谷之寒热，感则害于六腑"（《素问·阴阳应象大论》），"形寒寒饮则伤肺"（《灵枢·邪气脏腑病形》），因此，《灵枢·师传》指出"食饮者，热无灼灼，寒无沧沧"。

情绪失于调节如何导致衰老？

中医学认为，精神活动是脏腑活动的主宰，只有在人的情志活动和顺的情况下内脏功能才能平衡、协调，保持身体康健，若情志失调就会造成各种病变。中医理论认为，各个脏腑各有其一定的情志活动，《素问·阴阳应象大论》曰："人有五脏化五气，以生喜怒悲忧恐。"心"在志为喜"，肝"在志为怒"，脾"在志为思"，肺"在志为忧"，肾"在志为恐"。在一般情况下，这是人体正常的精神情志活动。若七情太过或太急，则可成为致病因素，引起人体气机失常，《素问·举痛论》曰："余知百病生于气也，怒则气上，喜则气缓，悲则气消，恐则气下……惊则气乱……思则气结。"说明了七情过极，超过机体心理生理调节能力，就会引起气血不和，阴阳失调，脏腑功能紊乱，导致早衰。

禀赋、体质与衰老有什么关系？

中医学很早就认识到人的寿命与禀赋渥薄和体质强弱相关。所谓禀赋主要是指遗传因素，而体质，则是人体在遗传性和获得性基础上表现出来的功能和形态上相对稳定的固有特性。《灵枢·阴阳二十五人》指出："火形之人……不寿暴死。"其"不寿"的原因很可能是受其体质因素中劣性遗传因子的影响。《灵枢·天年》记载："黄帝问曰：愿闻人之始生，何气筑为基？何立而为楯？……岐伯曰：以母为基，以父为楯。"王充在《论衡·气寿》中更是明确指出："强寿弱夭，谓禀气渥薄也……夫禀气渥则体强，体强则其命长；气薄则其体弱，体弱则命短。"

气候条件和地理环境对衰老的影响有哪些？

人的寿命与气候条件和地理环境有很大关系。自然界的风、寒、暑、湿、燥、火发生反常时就会成为致病的"六淫"，常常导致人体发生疾病。《灵枢·百病始生》曰："夫百病之始生也，皆生于风雨寒暑，清湿喜怒。"对"虚邪贼风"，应"避之有时"，并根据四时春夏秋冬不同气候的变化，"春夏养阳""秋冬养阴"。

地理环境对人体寿命的影响在《黄帝内经》中亦有所论述，《素问·五常政大论》中载"高者其气寿，下者其气夭"。高，指空气清新、气候较冷的高山地区；下，指炎热潮湿的低洼地区。因为"高者气寒"，植物生长较慢，生长期长，寿命也就长；而"下者气热"，植物生长较快，寿命相对短一些。

第三节
却 老

中医延缓衰老的原则是什么？

未病先防，未老先养。未病先防的思想是中医学的重要理论之一，《素问·四气调神大论》指出："是故圣人不治已病治未病，不治已乱治未乱，此之谓也。夫病已成而后药之，乱已成而后治之，譬犹渴而穿井，斗而铸锥，不亦晚乎！"这一"治未病"思想，对于养生抗老具有重大指导意义。张仲景继承《黄帝内经》这一学术思想，提出了"养慎"观点，认为内调饮食，导引吐纳，勿令房劳过度以养元气，外避寒暑，顺应四时以慎风邪，即可得百年之寿命。

广义来看，中医学所有养生防老方法都是以预防疾病、保健益寿为目的的。如起居调摄方面，《黄帝内经》强调对"风雨寒暑"等"虚邪贼风"要"避之有时"；饮食卫生方面，张仲景在《金匮要略》中专辟有《禽兽鱼虫禁忌并治》，强调预防食物中毒。孙思邈则在其著作中记载了用动物肝脏来预防夜盲症，用羊靥（甲状腺）和海带来预防地方性甲状腺肿。《素问·刺法论》曰："是故刺法有全神养真之旨，补法有修真之道，非治疾也。"开后世针刺或艾灸（如灸足三里、三阴交、气海、关元、中脘等穴位）养生的先河。因此中医养生学的指导思想应该是未老先养。

众所周知，人体生命的全过程可分为生、长、壮、老、已几个阶段，那么养老则不应当在进入老年期才开始实行，中医养生不但要养老，还应当养幼、养长，具体来说应包括受精、怀胎、分娩、哺育、养幼、养长、养老等内容。在这些方面，中医学有很多理论和实践经验，如重视优生、讲究胎教、爱护少儿健康、注重中年养生等。可以说，只有讲究养幼、养长，养老抗衰才会收到事半功倍的效果。

中医延缓衰老的方法有哪些？

中医延缓衰老的方法大致包括三个方面：一是日常调理、生活有节；二是自我锻炼、持之以恒；三是药食相兼、针灸相配。

延缓衰老的日常调理包括哪些方面？

遵循生活规律，注重日常生活如饮食、起居、睡眠、劳动及精神等方面的调养，对延缓衰老有重要作用。中医养生学强调食饮有节、起居适宜、心神舒畅，在长期的医疗保健实践中形成了一套行之有效的养生方法，如四时养生法、起居养生法、饮食养生法、睡眠养生法、精神养生法等。

中医学延缓衰老的自我锻炼方法有哪些？

中医学自我锻炼方法包括功法养生、按摩等。近代所谓的气功，源于古代的导引、吐纳等锻炼方法，关键在于调身、调心、调息。中国气功的历史悠久，流派纷呈，主要分为静功和动功两大类。导引也是中国古代形成的一种独特的强身延年功法，其主要作用是"导气令和，引体令柔"，使人体精力充盈、血脉流通。有的以调息引气为主，有的以运动肢体为主，如五禽戏、八段锦、易筋经、太极拳等。保健按摩在中国也由来已久，其主要作用是疏通血脉、调和气血，加强脏腑功能，祛除各种病邪。具体可分为头面按摩、全身按摩、穴位按摩等多种。上述方法是中医学特有的养生之道，可使人体排除内外干扰，形神合一地处于最佳状态，祛病防老延年。对个人来说，不需要掌握全部方法，选择一种自身适宜的方法，坚持锻炼，持之以恒，就能获益。

其他延缓衰老的方法有哪些？

药养：在中医历代文献中，不时可见到许多药物和方剂有"益气轻身""不老增年""延年益寿"等作用的记载，这些都属于药养范畴。近几年来，对具有抗衰老作用的中药和方剂，尤其是补肾类、健脾益气类、活血类等进行了重点研究，并从免疫，代谢，调整神经系统、内分泌和内脏功能，抗感染和调节微量元素等方面初步揭示了中药的抗衰老机制。

食养：古人认为"药食同源""药补不如食补"，张子和更是提出"养生当论食补"的观点。食疗是食补的主要形式，食疗方一般由食物和药物组成，取药物之性，用食物之味，食借药力，药助食攻，二者相辅相成，不同程度地提高机体免疫力，增强机体的生理功能，具有强身延年之功。

此外，还有针刺保健、养生灸、脐疗法、药枕疗法等许多行之有效、简单实用的方法。

第四节
至贵三宝

三宝的含义是什么？

"三宝"有多种含义。《老子》曰："吾有三宝，持而宝之，一曰慈，二曰俭，三曰不敢为天下先。"《孟子·尽心下》曰："诸侯之宝三：土地、人民、政事。"佛教所谓的三宝则指佛、法、僧。道家则认为精、气、神为内三宝，耳、目、口鼻为外三宝。而中医学所说的三宝主要是指精、气、神，对一个健康的人来说，这三者缺一不可，养生的精髓就在于调养这三种人体生命活动的基本物质。

"精"与生命活动的关系是什么？

形体是生命存在的基础，精是构成形体和形体赖以生长发育的物质，是构成生命的本源物质。《素问·金匮真言论》云"夫精者，身之本也"，《灵枢·决气》指出"两神相搏，合而成形，常先身生，是谓精"，《灵枢·经脉》指出"人始生，先成精，精成而脑髓生"，说明精是生命的原始物质，当男女之精结合后，在母体内形成胚胎，构成身形而产生生命。此精禀受于父母，与生俱来，故称为先天之精。其具有生殖繁衍作用，因而谓之生身之本。

精不仅是构成形体、产生生命的原始物质，也是维持生命活动、促进人体生长发育的基本物质。《医宗必读》曰："一有此身，必资谷气，谷入于胃，洒陈于六腑而气至，和调于五脏而血生，而人资之以为生者也。"人出生后不断从外界摄取水谷，在脾胃的作用下化生为水谷之精，输布于全身，营养脏腑官窍，筋骨肌肉，充养脑髓，促进生长发育，维持生命活动，此称为后天之精。后天之精藏于肾，肾精随着年龄渐盛而衰。从幼年始肾中精气渐充，出现齿更发长的生长变化；青春期精气充盛，生殖功能成熟，脑髓盈满，头脑清晰，思维敏捷，耳目聪明，肌肉丰满，毛发浓密，身体盛壮；老年期，精衰而致天癸竭，男子精少，女子经绝，形坏无子，发堕齿槁，面焦骨枯，耳目失聪，各方面的功能均衰减。因此，精与人体生、长、壮、老、已关系密切，是维持生命活动不息的本源物质。

"气"与生命活动的关系是什么？

气原属于哲学范畴，古代哲学家认为宇宙一切事物都是气的运动变化产生的。《周易·系辞》曰："天地氤氲，万物化生。"当"气"的概念被引入医学领域后，便用来解释人的生命活动。《素问·宝命全形论》指出："天地合气，命之曰人。"中医学认为人的生命活动是由气的运动变化产生的，气的运动形式不外乎升降出入。《素问·六微旨大论》曰："出入废，则神机化灭；升降息，则气立孤危。故非出入，则无以生长壮老已；非升降，则无以生长化收藏。是以升降出入，无器不有。"从生命伊始，气无时无刻不在进行升降出入运动，人体的呼吸、消化、吸收、视听、言行等都是通过气的升降出入运动而产生。气机升降不止，出入不息，互相配合，才能吸清呼浊，升清降浊，不断进行新陈代谢，维持生命活动。因此，气化是生命存在的特征。气化是通过气的升降出入运动而实现的，气有质无形，活动力很强，无处不在，通过升降出入运动而产生生命动力，激发维持脏腑组织的功能活动，不断进行气化作用，从而产生生命现象。因此，气是生命活动的原动力。

"神"与生命活动的关系是什么？

神有广义和狭义之分。中医学的神既指人的精神意识思维活动，又概括了复杂的生命形象，是一切生命活动的主宰者。神依附于形体而存在，随形体发育从无到有，从弱到强，形神合一即谓之人。《灵枢·天年》曰："血气已和，荣卫已通，五脏已成，神气舍心，魂魄毕具，乃成为人。"神是生命活动的外在表现，又主宰着一切生命活动，唯有神在，才能有人的一切的生命活动现象，故李东垣《脾胃论·省言箴》曰"积气以成精，积精以全神"，只有精充、气足、神全才能健康长寿。历代养生家都十分注重养神，如"得神者昌，失神者亡""太上养神，其次养形"。

"三宝"的相互关系是什么？

精是产生神的基础，气是化精之动力，神是精气的外在表现，寓于精气之中又为精气之主，三者缺一不可，均是人体生命活动的根本。故《类证治裁》指出"人身所宝，惟精气神，神生于气，气生于精，精化气，气化神，故精者身之本，气者神之主，形者神之宅也"。

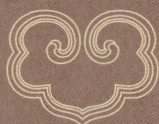

第三章

养　形

第一节
起居有常

一、顺应节律

为何要起居有常？

从天体的运动变迁，到人体的生命活动，都有其内在节律。中医学对此早有认识，认为人体气血受日月星辰、四时的影响而发生周期性的盛衰，故养生也应该起居有常，顺应阴阳变化。

起居有常应做到哪些？

第一，起居有常要顺应生命的节律，包括日节律、四时节律、五运六气变化节律等方面；第二，应保持合理睡眠；第三，应注重形体调护。

如何顺应一日之阴阳？

《素问·生气通天论》曰："阳气者，一日而主外，平旦人气生，日中而阳气隆，日西而阳气已虚，气门乃闭。是故暮而收拒，无扰筋骨，无见雾露，反此三时，形乃困薄。"说明一日之内阳气以中午最盛，到傍晚阳气已衰，人的起居要顺应这种变化，日出而作，日落而息，不然容易导致身体受损。

如何顺应四时之阴阳？

中医学认为，人生活在自然界中，与自然息息相关，人的起居只有顺应四时之阴阳变化，才能身体康健。四时节律就是春生、夏长、秋收、冬藏的规律。《素问·四气调神大论》曰："夫四时阴阳者，万物之根本也，所以圣人春夏养阳，秋冬养阴，以从其根，故与万物沉浮于生长之门；逆其根，则伐其本，坏其真也。故阴阳四时者，万物之始终也，死生之本也，逆之则灾害生，从之则苛疾不起，是谓得道。"强调四时阴阳变化对人体有极大的影响，起居顺应这种变化规律就健康，若违反这种规律变化，就会疾病丛生，所以提出了"春夏养阳，秋冬养阴"的总原则，在具体做法上，主张春季应该"夜卧早起，广步于庭"，夏季应"夜卧早起，无厌于日"，秋季应"早卧早起，与鸡俱兴"，冬季应"早卧晚起，必待日光"。

如何顺应年气的变化？

《素问·六元正纪大论》曰："先立其年以明其气，金木水火土运行之数，寒暑燥湿风火临郁之化，则天道可见，民气可调。"意谓根据中医五运六气学说，可测知每一年的气候变化规律和对人体的影响，人们可据此采取针对性的防治和养生措施。比如，当降水偏多之年，水湿流行，空气潮湿，人体易受湿邪侵袭，起居方面应注意防湿，甚至可用饮食（如多食辛温类食物）和药物（相对多用一些芳香走窜之品）来加以对抗。

二、劳逸适度

什么是劳，什么是逸？

　　劳和逸之间是一种相互对立、相互协调的辩证统一关系，二者都是人体的生理需要。中医学认为，劳包含形劳、神劳和房劳。逸，是指安逸。劳和逸是相对的，过度疲劳会损伤身体，过度安逸也会致病。人们在日常生活中应当做到有劳有逸，有张有弛。

　　经常合理地进行体力劳动和脑力劳动有利于畅通气血，活动筋骨，增强新陈代谢，健脑强身。一些有意义的劳动还能陶冶情操，开阔胸怀，从而保持旺盛的精力和愉快的情绪，增强体质，防止疾病发生。但劳动必须适度，尤其老年人从事脑力劳动和体力劳动，切勿过度疲劳，否则会引起疾病。

　　但也不能过于安逸，中医学认为"凡身体不可太逸，太逸则气血不畅，最易生病"。在日常生活中，如果不参加体育锻炼，四肢不勤，饱食终日，无所用心，就会引起气血不畅，筋骨脆弱，脾胃消化功能减退，食欲不振，身体软弱无力，抵抗力下降等。

劳而太过有哪些危害？

　　中医学认为劳而不可太过，劳役过度则内伤脏腑，正如《素问·宣明五气》中所说五劳所伤，即"久视伤血，久卧伤气，久坐伤肉，久立伤骨，久行伤筋"。所谓五劳，乃是人们平日里最为常见的五种不良的生活习惯，它们会给人体五脏带来伤害，从而发生劳损性疾病。故古人常说，"积劳成疾""五劳最易伤身"。

　　中国东汉名医华佗曰"人体欲得劳动，但不当使极尔，动摇则谷气得消，血脉流通，病不得生，譬犹户枢不朽是也"（《后汉书》），认为一定量的劳作或运动对人体是有利的，只是不应该太过，太过就会对身体造成伤害。孙思邈亦提出"不知养性之术亦难以长生也。养性之道，常欲小劳，但莫大疲及强所不能堪耳"（《备急千金要方》），明确指出要想长生必须要懂得养生，而养生的重点在于"常欲小劳"，"小劳"的意思就是微微有一点疲劳。古人认为过于安逸不利于长寿，就像不流动的水会腐臭，砍下来的树木会生虫一样。

养生为何要提倡运动？

《吕氏春秋》曰："流水不腐，户枢不蠹，动也。形气亦然，形不动则精不流，精不流则气郁。"《医学入门》记载："终日屹屹端坐，最是生死，人徒知久行久立伤人，而不知久卧久坐之尤伤人也。"可见，古代养生学家都意识到了运动对于生命的重要意义。中医学认为运动可使人全身气血流通，经脉通畅，脏腑功能活动正常，从而有益于延年。

养生的运动项目有哪些？

古人在长期与疾病作斗争、追求长寿的实践中，总结和发明了许多带有浓厚民族色彩的强身运动方法。如春秋战国时期，人们仿照飞禽走兽的动作而创立了二禽戏（熊经鸟申）；至西汉产生了三禽戏（熊、鸟、猿）；华佗继承《庄子》"吐故纳新，熊经鸟申"的法则，创立了动形养生的五禽戏；晋代又增补了燕飞、蛇屈、兔惊、龟咽等新的项目；至唐代有了八段锦、十二段锦；宋代有了"坐功"；明代有了太极拳、少林武术等。

现今，适合于人类的健身项目多种多样，大致包括以下几种。传统健身法：包括气功、导引、保健按摩、武术等；近代锻炼法：包括散步、跑步、游泳、汽车、球类等；医疗体育：比如针对慢性阻塞性肺疾病、高血压等的专门性医疗康复运动；天然健身法：包括日光浴、冷水浴、矿泉浴、森林疗法、空气疗法等。选择运动种类时，应根据个人的具体情况，做到运动有度、早期开始、持之以恒、动静结合。

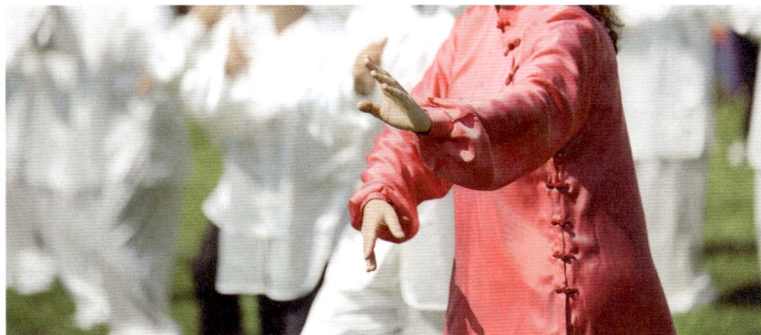

太极拳

如何做到动静结合？

古代养生学家，一方面主张动，另一方面又主张静，而且强调动静结合。以静为主者，首推老子和庄子。老子认为"静者躁君"（《道德经》），极力主张"致虚极，守静笃"，即要尽量排除杂念，坚守清静，"见素抱朴，少私寡欲"。庄子承老子之学，提出"抱神以静，形将自正，必清必静，无劳汝形，无摇汝精，乃可以长生"（《庄子·在宥》）。可见，以老、庄为代表的道家基本上是主张"清静无为"来养生的。《吕氏春秋》则提出"流水不腐，户枢不蠹"的著名观点，主张动以养生。至孔子时则提出"动静以义，喜怒以时，无害其性"的观点，主张动静结合（《孔子家语》）。

古代养生家们主张静是针对养神而言，认为内心清净、少私寡欲，就可使精神安藏于内，形体安居于外，实质就是以静"神"来养"形"，由此创立了很多静以养神的功法。但是，"静"只是运动的特殊形式，不是绝对的静止，老子、庄子等人在强调以静为主时，又创立了导引、吐纳等动态健身法。故最佳的养生法都是动静结合、形神兼养。

三、合理睡眠

何为睡眠养生？

睡眠养生指通过睡眠以消除疲劳，调节阴阳，恢复精神的一种养生方法。人生三分之一的时间都是在睡眠中度过的，充足良好的睡眠是保证身心健康的重要因素。对人体有利的睡眠首先必须是一个好的睡眠。

保持好睡眠的方法有哪些？

一是清净安眠法。睡前要清心寡欲，保持身心安静。在睡前 30 分钟不要思考问题，最好做一些松弛大脑紧张的活动，如散步、听轻音乐和戏曲，这些都有利于加快入睡。古人有"涪翁削官，投床鼻鼾"的说法，可见想要好的睡眠应当"先卧心，后卧眼"，心静神安方能入睡。

二是劳形安眠法。白天增加适当的体力活动，促使形体劳累，有助于睡眠，如睡前散步、练习八段锦等。古人有"轩辕毕泳，倚墙熟睡"的说法，可见适当的体力活动可以有助于睡眠。但睡前不可剧烈运动，正如古人所说"行则身劳，劳则思息"。

三是饮食安眠法。可适当选用一些有利于睡眠的药膳、药粥等改善睡眠。但切忌睡前饮食过饱，睡前亦不可饮用茶、酒、咖啡等刺激性饮料。

古人提倡的睡眠姿势是什么？

古人对睡眠姿势也相当讲究。《希夷睡诀》提倡：右侧卧，则屈右足；屈右臂，以手承头；伸左足，以手置于股间。左侧卧，与前相悖。

佛门规定右侧卧，名之曰"吉祥睡"，也是有科学道理的，因为人的心脏在左侧，如果左侧卧则可能压迫心脏。

中医学"子午流注"如何影响睡眠？

子午流注，是中医学的特色理论。子午是指时辰，流是流动，注是灌注。古代把一天划分为十二个时辰，即子、丑、寅、卯、辰、巳、午、未、申、酉、戌、亥，一个时辰相当于现在的两个小时，每个时辰都会有不同的经脉"值班"，即"肺寅大卯胃辰宫，脾巳心午小未中，申膀酉肾心包戌，亥焦子胆丑肝通"。人体内的气血也按照一定的节奏在各经脉间起伏流注，有盛有衰，首尾相衔，环环相扣，秩序井然。以子时为例，子时即夜里11点至凌晨1点，此时胆"值班"，胆经旺，中医理论认为"肝之余气，泄于明胆，聚而成精"。子时前入睡，晨起时头脑清晰、气色红润，没有黑眼圈。反之气色青黑，眼眶昏黑。因此，子时养生宜睡觉，忌熬夜、吃夜宵。

四、居处适宜

中医对居处地理环境与寿命关系的最早认识在何时？

《素问·五常政大论》曰："一州之气，生化寿夭不同，其故何也？岐伯曰：高下之理，地势使然也。崇高则阴气治之，污下则阳气治之，阳胜者先天，阴胜者后天，此地理之常，生化之道也。帝曰：其有寿夭乎？岐伯曰：高者其气寿，下者其气夭，地之小大异也，小者小异，大者大异。"此指居住在空气清新、气候寒冷的高山地区的人多长寿，而那些住在空气污浊、气候炎热的低洼地区的人则寿命相对较短一些。可见，中医学早在两千多年前就认识到了居处地理环境与寿命的关系，故《黄帝内经》提出养生应做到"和于阴阳，安于居处"。

地理环境如何影响人体健康？

《吕氏春秋·尽数》记载："轻水所，多秃与瘿人；重水所，多尰与躄人；甘水所，多好与美人；辛水所，多疽与痤人；苦水所，多尪与伛人。"意思是，久居雨露之地的人，容易脱发及长瘿瘤；久居井水之地的人多患脚肿及腿软；久居清泉之地的人，多容貌美好；久居温泉之地的人，易患疔疖之疾；久居盐碱清贫之地的人，易患鸡胸、驼背等病。可见，居住环境对健康非常重要。

住宅居所的哪些方面会对养生有影响？

一是住宅朝向。《宅经》指出，凡窗户朝向南、东南或西南方向的，室内采光就好。住宅朝向不仅影响采光，还可影响室内通风。就中国大部分地区来说，住宅坐北朝南是比较合理的，可充分利用太阳的光照，空气流通，冬暖夏凉。

二是住宅位置。居室择地，属于"看风水"的内容之一，早期并不是医家的事情，而是阴阳（堪舆）家的事。医家只是针对人体健康的需要，提出一些原则性的建议。如孙思邈在《千金翼方》中载"择地"，认为山林深处，宁静清秀，是建房的好环境，并强调"地势好亦居者安"。在有条件的农村，应该把住房建筑在那些依山傍水的地方，因为依山，冬季山上的树木可挡风避沙御寒；夏季茂密的树木可减少阳光辐射，吸收热量，调节气温，还能减轻和消除噪声，保持环境幽静。傍水则清澈流水可清除浊气。

三是美化环境。美化居住环境有利于健康长寿。《地新书》指出，住宅区应广种树木，四周栽竹，令青翠郁然，使人感到清新四溢，生机勃勃。《老老恒言》提倡在"院中植花木数十种，不求名种异卉"，四时不绝便佳，"阶前大缸贮水，养金鱼数尾"，并"事事不妨身亲之"，既美化了环境，锻炼了身体，又颐养了身心。有条件者可在房前屋后植树培草，使苍松翠柏，郁郁葱葱，绿树成荫。对于生活在现代都市中的城市居民来说，应因地制宜，充分利用阳台、窗台，采用盆花和攀缘类花草，青藤蔓绕，群花争艳，亦可使绿色常留身边。

如何选择居室？

居室是人们最重要的活动场所，人类几乎有一半以上的时间在此度过。对居室的要求，古人认为居室既不宜太高，也不能过矮，应该是宽敞适中，《天隐子》言"阴阳适中，明暗各半。屋无高，高则阳盛而明多，屋无卑，卑则阴盛而暗多"。房子不能太高，太高了就会日照太强且光线太亮；房子也不能太矮，太矮了则日照不够而光线太暗。从现代的观点来看，居室应该有良好的日照，居室高度应满足采光的要求和空气自然的流通，室高以 3 米左右为适，室内要温暖舒适、光线充足、通风良好、不可潮湿。对老年人的居室还另有讲究，《养老奉亲书》指出：老人居住的寝室，必须雅静清洁，夏天应虚敞，冬天应温暖致密；老人睡的床铺应当稳固，要比一般人用的床低一点，床的三边应有栏，床上的被褥、垫子一定要平整柔软；如有条件，老年人床上应夏挂纱幔，冬挂布帐，既防蚊虫叮咬，又可挡风避寒。

养生应如何美化居室？

　　优美舒适的居室对人的心理、生理都有良好的影响，居室美化没有具体的标准，总的原则是根据自己的情趣、爱好来布置房间。居室美化，应注意不要过于奢华，《备急千金要方》曰："至于居处，不得绮糜华丽，令人贪婪无厌，乃患害之源。但令雅素净洁，无风雨暑湿为佳。"认为居室内部的设置不用过分华丽奢侈，这种设置只能使人增长物欲的贪婪之心，是导致祸害的根源。居室清淡雅致、朴素干净，能够遮风挡雨、避暑免湿就是最好的。此外，可根据房间大小、个人爱好、经济适用等，摆上几盆花，养养鸟，喂喂鱼，或自己动手做几个小盆景，或挂上几幅名人字画，使人怡情养性，乐在其中。至于居室家具的摆放，应以整齐、实用、和谐，有利于休息和活动为原则。

第二节
法于阴阳

一、春季摄生

春季有什么气候特点？

《黄帝内经》曰："春三月，此谓发陈，天地俱生，万物以荣；夜卧早起，广步于庭，被发缓形，以使志生；生而勿杀，予而勿夺，赏而勿罚，此春气之应，养生之道也。逆之则伤肝，夏为寒变，奉长者少。"

春季三个月，始于立春止于立夏，春天是万物生发的季节，春归大地，冰雪消融，阳气升发，万物复苏，蛰虫活动，大地一派生机，万物欣欣向荣。人体阳气也顺其自然，向上向外疏发。但是春季气候也常变化，如乍暖还寒等。

春季如何养神？

春季万物勃发，养神应合于大自然的蓬勃生机，春应于肝，肝喜调达疏泄，恶于抑郁，因此，春季应保持心胸开阔，情绪乐观，不要烦恼生气。在风和日丽的春天，人们不要守舍不出，可以踏青问柳、游山戏水、观花赏泉，陶冶情操，以使自己精神愉快、心情舒畅，与自然融为一体。

春季如何调养起居？

春季气候渐暖，人体各系统的活动加强，使各器官的负荷增加，产生身体困乏的感觉，即民间所说的"春困"，为适应这种变化，应该晚睡早起，披散长发，舒展身体，漫步庭院。同时，春季气候多变，易寒易暖，要注意防风御寒，养阳敛阴，衣着方面"不可顿去寒衣……时备夹衣，遇暖易之，一重渐减一重，不可暴去"。民间有"春捂秋冻"的说法，确为经验之谈。春季又是极适合锻炼身体的季节，春光明媚，空气清新，万紫千红，生机盎然，若是能"闻鸡起舞"，实有利于人体吐故纳新，练气保精健体，既怡情养性，又锻炼形体。

春季如何进行饮食调养？

春季阳气升发，人体功能也处于旺盛之时，饮食宜选辛、甘、温之品，辛甘之品为阳，可助春阳之初发，温食有利于护阳，但应忌酸涩、油腻之物，肝亢于春，肝木过旺可克制脾土，故《备急千金要方》指出春日饮食宜"省酸增甘，以养脾气"，《摄生消息论》曰"饮酒不可过多，米面团饼，不可多食，致伤脾胃，难以消化"。

春季如何进行服食养生？

春季阳气生发，万物苏醒，各种毒邪也容易传播，如春季多发感冒、流感、上呼吸道炎症、流行性脑脊髓膜炎、麻疹等疾病，除积极治疗外，应注意空气消毒，在室内用艾叶加食醋熏蒸，可预防流感，同时内服中药板蓝根、贯众、甘草等，可起到预防作用。春季也是许多慢性疾病的发作期，如心脑血管疾病、过敏性哮喘等，除治疗外，中医还主张以预防为主，如《千金翼方》指出"凡人春服小续命汤五剂，及诸补散各一剂"能健身防病；《寿世秘典》亦云"三月采桃花浸酒饮之，能除百病，益颜色"等，这些都是具有一定意义的养生方法。

二、夏季摄生

夏季有什么气候特点？

《黄帝内经》曰："夏三月，此谓蕃秀，天地气交，万物华实，夜卧早起，无厌于日，使志无怒，使华英成秀，使气得泄，若所爱在外，此夏气之应，养长之道也。逆之则伤心，秋为痎疟，奉收者少，冬至重病。"

夏季三个月，始于立夏止于立秋。夏季是万物繁荣秀丽的季节，天阳下降，地热上蒸，天地阴阳之气上下交合，万物开始结果。夏季气候炎热，人体阳气也非常旺盛。

夏季如何养神？

夏季暑气当令，气候炎热，内应于心，阳气外发，伏阴在内，养神应做到内心安静、神清气和、快乐欢畅，切忌发怒，如《摄生消息论》曰："更宜调息静心，常如冰雪在心，炎热亦于吾心少减，不可以热为热更生热矣。"为适应夏季炎热的气候，可消暑避夏。总之，夏季养神要点是应尽量情绪外向，心胸开阔舒畅。

夏季如何调养起居？

夏季气候炎热，昼长夜短，可晚睡早起，适当午睡，以保存精力，夏季暑热偏胜，宜防曝晒，降室温，注意室内通风，谨防"中暑"，但又忌当风而眠，眠中风袭，尤其"老人当慎护，平居檐下、过廊、弄堂、破窗皆不可纳凉，此等所在虽凉，贼风中人最暴，惟宜虚堂净室，水亭木阴，洁净空敞之处，自然清凉"(《摄生消息论》)。衣着要选择浅色、宽大、透气性好的衣料，暑天出汗多，要勤洗澡，衣服要常洗常换。夏季锻炼身体也不能放松，可选择在清晨或傍晚，到公园、湖滨、林木下，以散步、慢跑、太极拳、气功、游泳等运动量不太大的项目为主。

夏季如何进行饮食调养？

夏季气候炎热，应于心火。《金匮要略》指出"夏不食心"，即根据中医脏器食疗法中"以心补心"的观点，认为夏季心气旺盛，不宜再补。《饮膳正要》载有"夏气热，宜食菽以寒之"，主张以食物的冷热燥湿来适应四时的变化。《养生书》曰："夏至后秋分前，忌食肥腻饼、油酥之属，此等物与酒浆瓜果，极为相仿，夏月多疾以此。"指夏季不应食肥甘油腻难以消化之品，否则会导致疾病发生。夏季食物易腐烂变质，故应注意饮食卫生，预防肠道传染病的发生，《论语》有"色恶不食，臭恶不食，失饪不食，不时不食"的记载，《金匮要略》亦有"秽饭、馁肉、臭鱼，食之皆伤人"的记载。

夏季如何进行服食养生？

夏季易患中暑、泄泻等疾病，中医学也主张用药物来预防疾病。如饮用绿豆汤、黄芪水，可清暑益气，生津止渴。《证治要诀》还主张常服荷叶粥，均有防暑作用。小满至小暑间多发暑病，可用麦冬、金银花、连翘、五味子、党参、茯苓、甘草煎水内服预防；大暑至白露易患湿病，可用白扁豆、薏苡仁、广藿香、生地黄等煎水内服预防。此外，对于一些冬季常发或加重的慢性疾病，如肺气肿、哮喘、腹泻等，中医学提倡"冬病夏治"，可起到较理想的防病治病的作用。

三、秋季摄生

秋季有什么气候特点？

《黄帝内经》曰："秋三月，此谓容平。天气以急，地气以明，早卧早起，与鸡俱兴，使志安宁，以缓秋刑，收敛神气，使秋气平，无外其志，使肺气清，此秋气之应，养收之道也。逆之则伤肺，冬为飧泄，奉藏者少。"

秋季三个月，始于立秋止于立冬。秋天是万物成熟、硕果累累的收获时节，时至秋令，天地间阳气日退，阴寒渐生，气候渐渐转凉，早晚气候变化很大，且常有冷空气袭击。阳气渐收，阴气渐长，景物也逐渐处于萧条状态，人体阳气也随之内收。

秋季如何养神？

秋季秋高气爽，气候渐凉，秋风劲疾，地气清肃，众生收杀，易使人产生悲伤忧愁之感。秋应于肺，悲忧最易伤肺，因此养神要做到内心宁静，神志安宁，心情舒畅，不要悲伤忧思，可以登高赏菊，观看红叶，以悦情志。

秋季如何调养起居？

秋季应"早卧早起，与鸡俱兴"，早睡以顺应阴精的收敛，早起以适应阳气的舒达。秋季气候特点是干燥，空气中湿度小、风力大，常易使人皮肤干燥，居室内应保持一定的湿度，并注意补充体内的水分，避免大汗淋漓以伤津液。秋季气温多变，早晚温差较大，应注意随时增减衣着。秋季也是锻炼的大好时机，秋季锻炼，可以静功为主，如内气功、意守功等，还可针对秋燥易伤肺的特点，用"叩齿""舌抵上腭""咽津""鼓呵"等方法养生，还可适当配合动功，如五禽戏、八段锦、太极拳等。另外，秋季可逐步做冷水浴等抗寒耐冻方面的锻炼。

秋季如何进行饮食调养？

秋季饮食调理的指导思想是防燥护阴、滋肾润肺，以"少辛增酸"为原则，《金匮要略》指出"秋不食肺"，因秋季肺气偏旺，不宜再补。《饮膳正要》曰："秋气燥，宜食麻以润其燥。"故应少食椒、葱、薤、蒜等辛燥之品，多进食芝麻、糯米、蜂蜜、甘蔗、菠菜、乳品等柔润之物，老人还可晨起食粥来益胃生津。《医学入门》载："盖晨起食粥，推陈致新，利膈养胃，生津液，令人一日清爽，所补不小。"百合莲子粥、银耳冰糖粥、红枣糯米粥、鲜生地汁粥、黑芝麻粥等均是益阴养胃且可久服多服的秋令佳品。

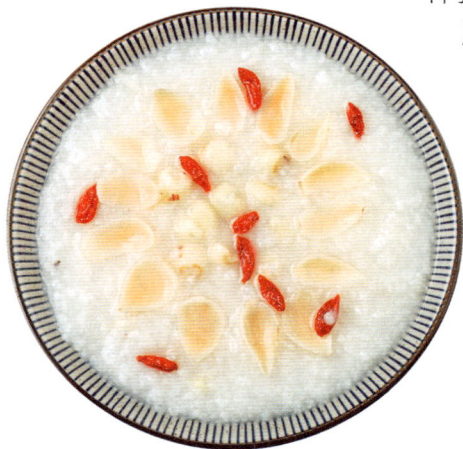

百合莲子粥

秋季如何进行服食养生？

根据秋季的气候特点，平时可服用人参、沙参、麦冬、百合、杏仁、川贝母、胖大海等具有益气滋阴、宣肺化痰功效的中药调养；秋分至立冬易发燥病，可用生地黄、百合、党参、蜂蜜、麦冬、甘草等内服，以防秋燥。

四、冬季摄生

冬季有什么气候特点？

《黄帝内经》曰："冬三月，此谓闭藏。水冰地坼，勿扰乎阳，早卧晚起，必待日光，使志若伏若匿，若有私意，若已有得，去寒就温，无泄皮肤，使气亟夺，此冬气之应，养藏之道也。逆之则伤肾，春为痿厥，奉生者少。"

冬季三个月，始于立冬止于立春。冬季是万物闭藏的季节，阴气盛极，阳气潜伏，草木凋零，昆虫蛰伏，大地冰封，气候寒冷，时有寒潮，人体阳气潜藏。

冬季如何养神？

冬临大地，万物凋零，内应于肾，养神应注意安静，含而不露，不要烦扰自身潜伏的阳气，尤其要注意避寒保暖，以藏阳气，可以观赏雪景来怡情养性。

冬季如何调养起居？

冬季天寒地冻，养生原则应是避寒就暖、敛阳护阴。起居方面，要"早卧晚起，必待日光"，"冬防寒，又防风"（《理虚元鉴》），所以室内温度应保持温暖；衣着方面，应以温暖舒适、气血流通为原则。此外，冬季为闭藏之时，更应固密心志，保精养神，故中医学尤其重视在冬天节制房事，《遵生八笺》中指出"冬三月六气十八候，皆正养脏之令，人当闭精塞神，以厚敛藏"，古人甚至还主张房事应"春一夏二秋一冬无"，充分说明节制房事、固护阴精以应冬令的重要性。冬季亦应克服气候寒冷的困难，积极参加健身锻炼。

冬季如何进行饮食调养？

冬季养生指导思想为"保阴育阳"，饮食的原则是"少咸"。《饮膳正要》曰："冬气寒，宜食黍，以热性治其寒。"主张进热食，但需注意燥热之物应适可而止，以免内伏之阳气郁而化热，当然生冷之物更应忌食，可多食羊肉、龟、藕、木耳、胡麻等物。冬季菜味可适当味重一些，可多食胡萝卜、菠菜、豆芽等新鲜蔬菜。冬季活动量少，人体新陈代谢减慢，饮食不宜过饱，食后可摩腹以助食运。

冬季如何服食养生？

冬主闭藏，"冬藏精"，冬季是进补的好时机，但无论是食补还是药补，都应根据自身情况，在医生指导下进行，不可盲目进补。通常情况下，阳气偏虚者，食补以羊肉、鸡肉等为主，药补还可用人参、鹿茸、金匮肾气丸等方药；阴血偏虚者，食补可用鸭肉、鹅肉、猪肝、木耳等，药补可用阿胶、当归、枸杞子、六味地黄丸等。此外，体虚者不可大补、峻补，应当循序渐进。对于体质健康者，最好是用食补，在冬令时可行药补，且最好是清补、小补；对于体质衰弱者，可食补和药补并重。

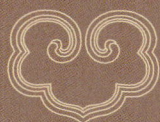

第四章

养 神

第一节
形神合一

什么是形？什么是神？

中医学认为，人体是由"形"和"神"组成。所谓"形"，指人的整个形体结构，包括五脏六腑、经络、四肢百骸等组织结构和气血津精等基本营养物质，是物质基础。所谓"神"，有广义和狭义之分。广义的神指整体生命活动现象，包括语言、眼神、肢体活动姿态及整个人体的形象等；狭义的神指中医学心所主的神志，包括人的精神、意识、情感等活动，是功能作用。

何谓"形神合一"？

张景岳在《类经》中指出："形者神之体，神者形之用；无神则形不可活，无形则神无以生。"又云："人禀天地阴阳之气以生，借血肉以成其形，一气周流于其中以成其神，形神俱备，乃为全体。""形神合一"是中医学的生命观，又称为"形与神俱"或"形神相印"，即形体与精神的统一。中医的"神"不仅主导人的精神活动，也主宰人的物质代谢和能量代谢。"神"虽由精气化生，但反过来支配精气活动，说明"形"与"神"相互依存、相互影响、密不可分。

如何做到"以神养形"？

神对整体功能起着主宰和调节作用，中医养生学家认为调神为第一要义，神的功能状态决定了养生的成败。《素问·灵兰秘典论》记载："心者，君主之官也，神明出焉。"《素问·调经论》说："心藏神。"中医学认为"神"是人体活动的主宰，神明的产生分属于五脏，但总统于心。因此，养神即养心，心神调养得当则"主明则下安，以此养生则寿，殁世不殆，以为天下则昌"；心神失养，则"主不明则十二官危，使道闭塞不通，形乃大伤，以为天下者，其宗大危"。三国时期养生家嵇康在《养生论》中也提出"修性以保神，安心以全身"的养生思想。综上可见，保养心神是养生保健的首要问题。

怎样才能做到"形神俱在"？

形神共养是中医学推崇的一种最高养生方法。《黄帝内经》明确提出了"形与神俱"的形神共养的观点，如《素问·上古天真论》曰："故能形与神俱，而尽终其天年，度百岁乃去。"并提出了"虚邪贼风，避之有时"的外避邪气以养形，以及"恬惔虚无，精神内守"的内养真气以充神的形神合养的方法。在《素问·四气调神大论》中更进一步记载了随着春夏秋冬四时不同气候来形神共养的健身法，如春三月，养形应该"夜卧早起，广步于庭，披发缓形"，以此来养神，从而达到"以使志生"。中医养生学历史悠久，源远流长，具体的养生方法多种多样，但归纳起来不外乎"养形"与"养神"两种，即所谓"守神全形"和"保形全神"，无论是"全形"还是"全神"，都是通过形神合养，使神旺形安，而尽终天年。

第二节
情志调摄

七情太过对人体的影响有哪些？

《素问·天元纪大论》云："人有五脏化五气，以生喜怒思忧恐。"中医学的情志即指喜、怒、忧、思、悲、惊、恐七种情绪，情志由五脏之气化生。因此，中医学认为，情志活动与内脏关系十分密切；过激的情志活动也可使内脏发生疾病。主要表现为：一是导致气机失常。如《素问·举痛论》云："百病生于气也，怒则气上，喜则气缓，悲则气消，恐则气下，寒则气收，炅则气泄，惊则气乱，劳则气耗，思则气结。"二是导致阴阳失调。《素问·疏五过论》云："暴怒伤阴，暴喜伤阳。厥气上行，满脉去形。"就是说生气大怒损伤人体之阴，过喜则耗伤阳气。《灵枢·百病始生》云："喜怒不节则伤脏，脏伤则病起于阴也。"认为喜怒如果没有节制会损伤五脏，五脏为阴，所以说脏伤则病起于阴。三是导致精血亏损。《医学入门》曰："暴喜动心不能主血。"意为过度喜悦会损伤心气。中医学认为心的功能之一是心主血，心气损伤的心不能主血，容易出现血虚、血瘀等血证。四是直接损伤脏腑。《素问·阴阳应象大论》云："怒伤肝，喜伤心，思伤脾，忧伤肺，恐伤肾。"比较形象地阐明了不同情志的过极对于相应脏腑的影响。五是出现系列症状。隋代巢元方《诸病源候论》云："怒气则上气不可忍，热上抢心，短气欲死，不得气息也。恚气则积聚在心下，不可饮食。忧气则不可极作，暮卧不安席。喜气即不可疾行，不能久立。愁气则喜忘不识人，置物四方，还取不得去处，若闻急即手足筋挛不举。"意为发怒的时候会有燥热、气短的感觉，怨气则容易累积在心下，容易吃不进食物，忧虑的情绪则导致失眠等。

如何调摄情志？

在情志调摄方面，总的来说要做到"和喜怒，调刚柔"。《灵枢·本神》曰："故智者之养生也，必顺四时而适寒暑，和喜怒而安居处，节阴阳而调刚柔。如是则僻邪不至，长生久视。"《钱公良测语》有"大喜不喜，大怒不怒，可以养心"一说。此外，《曾国藩家书》中有著名的"八本""三致祥"观点。"八本"，即"读古书以训诂为本，作诗文以声调为本，养亲以得欢心为本，养生以少恼怒为本，立身以不妄语为本，治家以不晏起为本，居官以不要钱为本，行军以不扰民为本"，其中"养生以少恼怒为本"讲的也是要和喜怒，调情志。"三致祥"，即孝致祥、勤致祥、恕致祥。他认为，孝顺父母、勤劳节俭、宽厚待人，是能够为家族带来祥瑞并且必须遵循的品行。

第三节
修心养性

修心养性为何如此重要？

中国古代养生医家素来注重心性修养，认为人处天地之间，其心态对于整体损益兴衰有着至关重要的作用。因此，古代养生家们特别强调养心、养性、养德。古人认为"养生首重养心"，养心是指修身养性，儒、释、道三家学问也都非常重视修身养性，重视心身双修、性命双修。儒家认为养心、修心、育心在"修身齐家治国平天下"中非常重要。《大学》云："物格而后知至，知至而后意诚，意诚而后心正，心正而后身修，身修而后家齐，家齐而后国治，国治而后天下平。"

如何做到修心养性？

在心性修养中，最重要的是要做到清心寡欲。《黄帝内经》认为"恬惔虚无，真气从之，精神内守，病安从来。是以志闲而少欲，心安而不惧，形劳而不倦"。孟子也提出相似的观点，认为"养心莫善于寡欲"。就是说在思想上要保持内心清净安宁，不贪求妄想，就可精神健旺，预防疾病。为了做到少私寡欲，古代先哲还主张"抑目静耳"，因目和耳是人体接触外界刺激的主要渠道，目清耳净则神气内守而心不劳，若目驰耳躁，则神气劳烦而心忧不宁。《千金翼方》指出"养老之要，耳无妄听，口无妄言，身无妄动，心无妄念，此皆有益老人也"。

古人还认为养性可以延命，只有在养生中注意养德，才能跻身仁寿之域。孔子在《中庸》里就明确指出"修身以道，修道以仁。大德必得大寿"。《大学》有言："富润屋，德润身。"《论语》云："知者乐，仁者寿。"明代高濂《遵生八笺》云："善养生者，养内；不善养生者，养外。外贪快乐，姿情好尚，务外则虚内矣。所谓养内者，使五脏安和，三焦守位，饮食得宜，世务不涉，是可长寿。"这从具体做法上给予了我们一些指导。明代医家龚廷贤在《寿世保元》中云："积善有功，常存阴德，可以延年。"凡此种种，古人认为这样能达到延年益寿目的。

气功如何指导心性修养？

有一种特殊形式的养心之术——气功。气功一词古已有之，晋代许逊著的《净明宗教录》中就有"气功阐微"之称，在晋以前的典籍中，道家称之为"吐纳""炼丹"，儒家称之为"正心""修身"，佛门称之为"参禅""止观""打坐""入定"，医生称之为"导引""摄生"，甚至太极拳等某些武术，只要以内功为基础，都属气功的范畴。气功主要通过调节姿势、锻炼呼吸、松弛身心、控制意识、有节律地运动身体等，使身心融为一体，以达到预定的锻炼目的。即通过内向性地运用意识，使自身的意识活动和生命活动相结合，增强机体生命活动、启发人体内在潜能，从而起到陶冶性情、开发智慧、防病治病、延年益寿作用。包括调身（调节姿势）、调息（调整呼吸）和调心（安定思想）三个方面。

何谓怡情十乐？

怡情畅神，要求把生活安排得丰富多彩，培养高雅的兴趣，陶冶高尚的情操，从而保持"常乐"的心境。徐春甫在《古今医统大全》中曰："凡人平生为性，各有好嗜之事，见则喜之。有好书画者，有好琴棋者，有好博弈者，有好珍奇者，有好药饵者，有好禽马者，有好古物者……使其喜爱玩悦不已。"《寿亲养老新书》载有"十乐"：读书义理、学法帖字、澄心静坐、益友清谈、小酌半醺、浇花种竹、听琴玩鹤、焚香煮茶、泛舟观山、寓意弈棋。清代画家高桐轩也有"十乐"：耕耘之乐、扫帚之乐、教子之乐、知足之乐、安居之乐、畅谈之乐、漫步之乐、沐浴之乐、高卧之乐、曝背之乐。

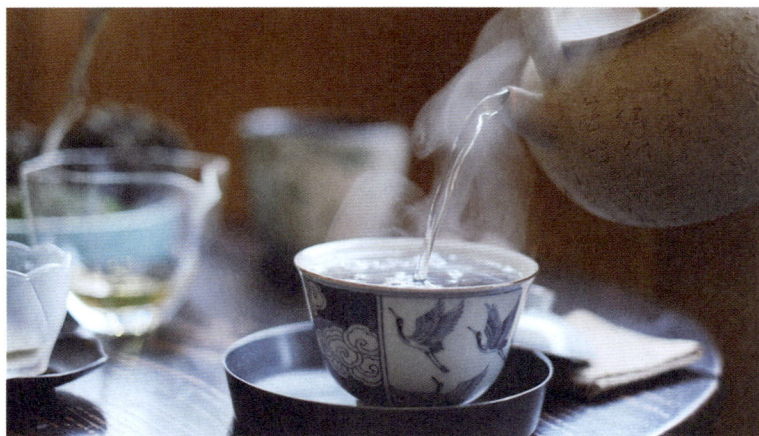

饮茶

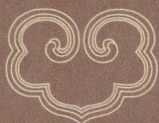

第五章

食　养

第一节
食养概述

何谓饮食养生？

饮食养生，又称食养，是在中医基本理论指导下，研究食物的性能，利用食物维护健康，延年益寿，或辅助药物防治疾病，预防疾病复发的养生方法。

饮食养生包括哪些内容？

饮食养生的内容，从历代文献记载和临床实际情况看，主要包括维护健康、防治疾病、愈后防复三个方面，以及饮食节制、饮食宜忌两种方法。

合理饮食，维护健康，又称"食养""食补"，是利用饮食营养机体、保持健康或增进健康的活动。《素问·五常政大论》载"谷肉果菜，食养尽之"，即"食养"概念的早期记载。

利用膳食，防治疾病，又称"食疗""食治"，指用饮食来治疗或辅助药物治疗疾病的活动。孙思邈在《备急千金要方·食治》云"食能排邪而安脏腑，悦神，爽志，以资血气"，体现了食疗祛邪与扶正两方面的作用。后又有食疗专著《食疗本草》等相继问世。

饮食调养，愈后防复，指利用合理的饮食节制和饮食宜忌，根据病情，辨证进食，从而使机体尽快康复，防止病情复发。《素问·热论》曰"病热少愈，食肉则复，多食则遗，此其禁也"，具体阐述了热病恢复阶段饮食调养的注意事项。

为何古代医家注重食药并重？

中国第一部药物专著《神农本草经》收载药物 365 种，其中很多药味既是药物又是食物。《周礼·天官》有"食医""疾医""疡医"之属，所设"食医"，即专职管理食物养生和饮食卫生的医生。《素问·五常政大论》指出，在疾病缓解后应"谷肉果菜，食养尽之"，以助病后健康恢复。《素问·脏气法时论》曰："五谷为养，五果为助，五畜为益，五菜为充，气味合而服之，以补精益气。"可见古人在治疗过程就主张食药并用。东汉医家张仲景采用不少食物以治病，如《伤寒论》和《金匮要略》记载的"猪肤汤"和"当归生姜羊肉汤"都是典型的食治专方。唐代孙思邈编著的《备急千金要方》和《千金翼方》分别立有"食治"专卷和"养老食疗"专篇，提出"夫为医者，当需先洞晓病源，知其所犯，以食治之；食疗不愈，然后命药"，并引用扁鹊语"安身之本必须于食，救急之道惟在于药，不知食宜者，不足以全生……有疾期先命食以疗之，食疗不愈然后命药"。

中国古代的食疗专著有哪些？

唐代孟诜所撰《食疗本草》是中国第一部食疗专著，集唐以前食疗之大成。唐代另一食疗专著是昝殷的《食医心鉴》，共收集食疗验方200余首，有羹、煎、粥、馄饨、饼、茶、酒等种类，尤其注重粥疗，载药粥57方，为后世药粥疗法奠定了基础。此后还出现了《饮膳正要》《寿亲养老新书》《食鉴本草》《随息居饮食谱》《饮食辨录》等食养专著，说明食养一直都很受人们的重视。元代《寿亲养老新书》曰："人若能知其食性，调而用之，则倍胜于药也。"可见食养是中医药学宝库中的重要组成部分，为中华民族的防治疾病、养生保健、烹调营养等方面都做出了贡献，是养生的重要方法之一。

食养不当有何危害？

历来有"药补不如食补"的说法，但食补并非人人皆可用，也不是有病即可施，《金匮要略》特别强调饮食不当对身体的影响，曰："凡饮食滋味，以养于身。食之有妨，反能为害……害则成疾，以此致危。"

第二节
辨证施膳

食养如何兼顾脾胃功能？

脾胃功能旺盛时，可根据疾病需要配合饮食营养，如体虚贫血严重者，可加强血肉有情之品以补养，适当地选择高蛋白类食物及动物肝脏以补血。若脾胃功能薄弱，食欲减退，脘腹作胀，便溏，苔厚腻，就不能强调"虚者补之"，饮食太过，反而增加脾胃负担，"虚不受补"者，宜清淡饮食，先调理脾胃，待脾胃功能恢复，再予以食补。

食养如何做到因人施膳？

《金匮要略》曰："羊肉其有宿热者，不可食之。""妇人妊娠，不可食兔肉……令子无声音。"这些虽尚待进一步研究，但说明食养必须因人而异。如公鸡、猪头肉等对一般人而言是有补益作用的，但素患肝阳头痛、头风者则不可服食，服用可诱发宿疾；又有个别特异禀质之人，食鱼、虾、蟹等可出现过敏反应，诱发荨麻疹、哮喘等病。

食养如何做到因地制宜？

《黄帝内经》指出东方之域为鱼盐之地，其民"食鱼而嗜咸""鱼者使人热中，盐者胜血"，其发病"皆为痈疡"（《素问·异法方宜论》），说明食养必须因地制宜。如冬季进补时，北方气候严寒，可选择大温大热之品进行食养，如羊肉、鹿肉等；而南方气候温和，宜选用甘温清补之品，如猪肉、鸡、鸭、鱼等。长期在水上作业之人或海边居住者，多湿邪内侵，食养时必须佐以健脾燥湿中药；而长期高空作业或居住在山区者，多燥邪相干，食养时须多用清宣凉润之品，如银耳、冰糖、梨、鳖、龟等。

食养如何做到因时施补？

古人食养非常注重因时施补，《千金食治·序论》曰："夏至以后，迄至秋分，必须慎肥腻、饼臛、酥油之属。"又曰："春七十二日，省酸增甘，以养脾气；夏七十二日，省苦增辛，以养肺气；秋七十二日，省辛增酸，以养肝气；冬七十二日，省咸增苦，以养心气；季月各十八日，省甘增咸，以养肾气。"可见四时节令变化，在食养方面应随之有所调整。又如夏令之时，年老体弱之人，由于适应能力减退，耐不得炎热酷暑，除注意避暑之外，可吃些清凉性的食养品，既可解热消暑，又能生津止渴，如绿豆粥、荷叶粥等；寒冬腊月，最易伤人阳气，老年人阳气不足，可适当吃一些温补性的食养品以温阳散寒，如羊肉粥、肉苁蓉粥等。

如何辨证施膳？

由于个人身体素质不同，生活习惯各异，病情证候有别，所表现出来的虚弱情况及疾病的性质也各有不同。因此，食养必须辨识寒热虚实、脏腑气血阴阳之亏损而辨证施膳，合理选用补气、补血、补阴、补阳、养心、养肝、养脾、养肺、养肾等食养品。如阴虚者宜清补，可用百合、龟甲、海参、银耳等；阳虚者宜温补，可用羊肉、鹿肉等。

食养的目的在于使机体"阴平阳秘"，调整机体脏腑的阴阳气血，使之趋于平衡。因此不可盲目地"气虚益气，血虚补血，阴亏养阴，阳虚壮阳"，因益气太过反可致气机壅滞，升降失常，养阴太过又可遏伤阳气，而致阴寒更重，所以益气勿忘补血，补血勿忘益气，养阴需佐温阳，温阳须固护阴液，如此方能阴阳气血平衡。

药膳是药物和食物结合，两者具有协同作用。食物和药物一样是禀受天地阴阳之气而生，两者均具有性、味、升降浮沉、归经，也称为药性和食性。因药性、食性不同，作用也就各异。在施膳前应根据食用者的病症、体质结合所处的地理环境、生活习惯以及季节的不同，正确地辨证选药组方或选食配膳，做到"组药有方、方必依法、定法有理，理必有据"，只有这样才能达到预期的目的。药膳形如食品，性同药品，药膳是药物以食物为载体，通过类似食物的烹调方法加工制作，使药物、食物共同发挥一定效用的一种物品。它既不同于一般的食品，也不同于一般药品，它和食物一样具有色、香、味等感官性状，又具有安全、无毒、有效的作用特点，两者结合，相互协同，达到药借食力、食助药攻的目的。

如何应用药膳？

中年人药膳应用原则：中年时期是身体由盛转衰的转折时期，脏腑器官功能逐渐衰退，特别是肾精逐渐亏虚，加之生活、工作压力较大，使阴血暗耗，脏腑功能衰退，出现头晕、心慌、乏力、记忆力下降、性功能障碍等，甚至出现早衰，这一时期的保健强身显得尤为重要。对更年期女性，用具有疏肝理气、滋阴补肾功效的药膳，长期应用有减轻更年期症状、健肤美容的效果。

老年人药膳应用原则：老年人各个脏腑的功能已经衰退，常出现以头昏心慌、气短乏力、失眠多梦、食欲不振、健忘耳鸣、性功能减退、便秘等为表现的气虚血少、肾精亏虚、脾虚津枯、气虚痰凝、气虚痰瘀等一系列虚证及本虚标实证。药膳宜选补精填髓、补益气血、壮腰健肾、益气活血类药物。

第三节
调和五味

食物的性味有哪些?

食物的"性",主要指"寒、热、温、凉"之性,"味",主要指"酸、苦、甘、辛、咸"之味。

如何利用食物之"性"进行食养?

药性的温热与寒凉是对立的两大属性,饮食养生的精髓就是利用食物的偏性纠正人体的偏性。中医治病的大法是"治寒以热,治热以寒",饮食调养的原则也是这样,热性体质的人或热证患者适宜吃寒性的食物而不宜吃热性的食物;寒性体质的人或寒证患者适宜吃热性食物而不宜吃寒性食物。

常见的热性食物有辣椒、花椒、姜、蒜、葱、酒、龙眼肉、羊肉、公鸡等,常见的寒性食物有绿豆、白萝卜、豆腐、荸荠、螃蟹、甲鱼、梨、柿子等。

如何利用食物之"酸"味进行食养?

"酸"味能收能涩。酸味药具有收敛固涩的作用,具体体现为止泻、敛汗、涩精、缩尿、止带、止血等制止人体阴液滑脱的作用,以及敛肺气而止咳嗽、收敛心神而安神等无形的作用。

酸味药还具有生津作用。三国时的著名故事"望梅止渴",就是利用酸味生津的作用。三伏天酷暑难耐,汗出如雨,体内津液大量散失,引起口渴尿少,民间常用的食疗方法就是喝酸梅汤,以生津开胃、消暑解渴、除烦安神。

酸味药可用于胃阴不足之口干舌燥、不思饮食、舌红少苔,或舌苔剥落等症,或津液耗伤、筋脉失养而致的筋脉拘挛、屈伸不利;还可用于体虚多汗、肺虚久咳、久泻肠滑、遗精滑精、尿频遗尿、崩带不止等。由于酸味药大多能收敛邪气,凡邪未尽之证均当慎用。

酸味膳食原料有山楂、乌梅、木瓜、石榴、苹果、草莓等。因为酸能收敛,多食也有一定副作用。唐代的《食疗本草》云石榴"久食损齿令黑",杨梅"不可多食,损人齿及筋也",可见酸味食物摄入过多对身体也有损伤。

如何利用食物之"苦"味进行食养?

"苦"味能泻、能燥、能坚,即具有清泄火热、泄降气逆、通泄大便、燥湿、坚阴（泻火存阴）等作用。一般来讲，苦味药多用于热证、火证、喘咳、呕恶、便秘、湿证、阴虚火旺等。因苦燥易伤阴津，阴津不足者不宜用。苦寒之药易伤伐脾胃阳气，用量过大，或服用过久，易致脾胃阳虚，食欲不振、大便稀溏，故素体脾虚者亦当慎用。

苦味膳食原料有杏仁、香橼、黄花菜、枸杞菜、苦瓜、莴笋、蒲公英、苦蓟、芹菜等。近年来，越来越多的人崇尚回归自然的生活方式，喜欢吃野菜的人越来越多，这些野菜大多味苦，能清热开胃，对容易上火的人非常有益。

中国人饮茶已有几千年历史，茶叶属于苦味饮品，其性兼寒，具有清利头目、下气消食、利大小肠等诸多功效，古人用茶叶治疗水泻，就是利用它燥湿利水的作用。当然，苦味吃太多也会伤胃，尤其是素体胃寒的人不宜多食。

如何利用食物之"甘"味进行食养？

"甘"味能缓能补，味道甘甜的食物具有补益、缓急的作用。日常生活中主食大多数是甘味，中医学认为甘味能入脾胃，甘与脾相对应，甘味食物如山药、大枣、莲子肉、薏米、白扁豆等可用来调补脾胃。调补脾胃的常用处方参苓白术散、资生丸中，就有很多药食同源的"甘"味中药。但甘能壅气，过食甘甜之味易导致饱胀闷满，不思饮食。

如何利用食物之"辛"味进行食养？

"辛"味能散能行，可行气健胃，散寒活血。具有辛味的食物有很多，如姜、葱、韭、酒、香菜、胡椒、花椒、桂皮、洋葱、茴香、萝卜等。辛味食物大多是热性的，民间习惯在腹部受凉时喝姜汤，即取其行气健胃的作用；外感初起时，喝葱白汤，即取其解表散寒作用；妇女产后喝黄酒、红糖水等，即取其散寒行气活血作用；川渝地区多潮湿，居民嗜食辣椒、花椒等辛辣食物，能有效祛除和抵御寒湿之气。

如何利用食物之"咸"味进行食养？

"咸"味能下、能软，即具有泻下通便，软坚散结的作用。咸味药多用于大便燥结、痰核、瘿瘤、癥瘕痞块等。

此外，《素问·宣明五气》还有"咸走血"之说。肾属水，咸入肾，心属火而主血，咸走血即以水胜火之意。如大青叶、玄参、紫草、青黛、白薇都具有咸味，均入血分，具有清热凉血解毒之功。《素问·至真要大论》又云："五味入胃，各归所喜攻……咸先入肾。"故不少入肾经的咸味药如海狗肾、蛤蚧等都具有良好的补肾作用。同时为了引药入肾，增强补肾作用，不少药物如知母、黄柏、杜仲等药用盐水炮制。

《黄帝内经》如何指导谷果菜肉搭配？

早在两千多年前，《素问·脏气法时论》就指出："五谷为养，五果为助，五畜为益，五菜为充，气味合而服之，以补精益气。"阐述了粮食、肉类、蔬菜、水果是饮食的主要组成，同时还说明了调配饮食的规律，即以粮食为主食，肉类为副食，蔬菜作为补充，水果作为辅助。

常见的谷类食物有哪些功效？

谷物自古以来就是中国人民的主要主食来源，《周礼》郑玄注"五谷"为"麻、黍、稷、麦、豆"。各种谷物的共同特点是性质比较平和，味甘，甘先入脾，因此长期食用这些主食可发挥重要的调养脾胃的作用。不同种类的谷物其性质亦有差别，中国唐代著名养生学家孙思邈在《备急千金要方》中详述了以下几类谷物。

粳米（大米），味辛、苦，平，无毒。主心烦，断下利，平胃气，长肌肉，温中。

糯米，味苦，温，无毒。温中，令人能食，多热，大便硬。

陈廪米，味咸、酸，微寒，无毒。除烦热，下气调胃，止泄利。

小麦，味甘，微寒，无毒。养肝气，去客热，止烦渴咽燥，利小便，止漏血唾血。

荞麦，味酸，微寒，无毒。食之难消，动大热风。其叶生食动刺风，令人身痒。黄帝云：作面和猪、羊肉热食之，不过八九顿，作热风，令人眉须落，又还生，仍稀少。泾邠以北，多患此疾。

薏苡仁，味甘，温，无毒。主筋拘挛，不可屈伸，久风湿痹下气。

生大豆，味甘，平，冷，无毒。生捣，淳酢和涂之，治一切毒肿，并止痛。煮汁冷服之，杀鬼毒，逐水胀，除胃中热，却风痹、伤中、淋露，下瘀血，散五脏结积内寒，杀乌头三建，解百药毒。

赤小豆，味甘、咸，平，冷，无毒。下水肿，排脓血。一名赤豆。不可久服，令人枯燥。

青小豆，味甘、咸，温、平，涩，无毒。主寒热，热中，消渴；止泄利，利小便，除吐逆、卒澼、下腹胀满。

大豆豉，味苦、甘，寒，涩，无毒。主伤寒头痛，寒热，辟瘴气恶毒，烦躁满闷，虚劳喘吸，两脚疼冷，杀六畜胎子诸毒。

常见的蔬菜有哪些功效？

冬瓜，甘、淡，微寒。益气生津，清热利水。

黄瓜，甘，寒。清热止渴，利水解毒。

南瓜，甘，温。补中益气，利水解毒，杀虫。

芹菜叶，苦，微寒。清热利湿，降压降脂。

韭菜，辛，温。温阳补虚，行气理血。

番茄，甘、酸，微寒。健脾消食，生津止渴，清热利尿，凉血平肝。

胡萝卜，甘，平。益气生血，健胃消食，明目养肝。

萝卜，辛，凉。宽中下气，化痰消积，清热解毒，凉血生津。

茄子，甘，寒。清热和血，散瘀消肿。

竹笋，苦，微寒。利五脏，通经脉，强筋骨，宽胸利气。

马铃薯，甘，平。健脾益气，和胃调中。

藕，甘，寒。健脾开胃，润肺生津，凉血清热。

海带，咸，寒。消痰软坚，清热利水。

香菇，甘，平。补气健脾，和胃益肾。

木耳，甘，平。益气补脑，润肺生津，止血凉血。

辣椒，辛，热。温中散寒，开胃消食，除湿发汗。

大蒜，辛，温。温中散寒，行气消积，解毒杀虫。

大葱，辛，温。发表散寒，通阳利窍。

常见的水果有哪些功效？

西瓜，甘，寒。清热解暑，生津利尿。

桃，甘、酸，温。益气生津，活血消积，润肠通便。

梨，甘、微酸，寒。养阴生津，润肺止咳，清热化痰。

李，甘、酸，平。清热生津，利水行瘀。

杏，酸、甘，温。生津止渴，润肺定喘。

栗子，甘，温。补骨强筋，健脾益气，活血止血。

常见的肉类有哪些功效？

猪肉，甘、咸，平。益气养血，滋阴润燥。可"丰肌体，泽皮肤，润肠胃，生津液"，但多食则生痰生湿，动风助热。

牛肉，甘，平，偏温。补脾益气，养精血，强筋骨。

羊肉，甘，温。补气养血，温肾祛寒。

羊肉、鹿肉、雄鸡，性偏温热，宜在冬天食用。

雌鸡，性平，多用于产妇和失血患者。

鸭肉，性寒，可补虚除热。

第四节
药膳养生

药膳的原料有哪些？

药膳的原料，主要是指进行食养所需要的食物与中药，一般中药多为滋补类中药，而食物种类繁多，有动物类、植物类、禽蛋类等。

养气、血、阴、阳常用的中药：人参、党参、黄芪、白术、怀山药、茯苓、当归、阿胶、白芍、熟地黄、桃仁、枸杞子、贝母、天冬、百合、竹叶、麦冬、沙参、冬虫夏草、干姜、肉苁蓉、灵芝等。

养气、血、阴、阳常用的食物：鸡肉、鸭肉、鱼肉、兔肉、羊肉、海参、牛肉、猪肝、萝卜、燕窝、甲鱼、小麦、绿豆、鸽蛋、鸡蛋、西瓜、雪梨、猪肚、猪肘、鹿肉等。

养心、肝、脾、肺、肾常用的中药：龙眼肉、酸枣仁、党参、当归、柏子仁、百合、枸杞子、菊花、木贼、桑椹、白芍、怀山药、砂仁、豆蔻、莲子、大枣、山楂、神曲、白术、扁豆、芡实、麦冬、沙参、冬虫夏草、川贝母、银杏、核桃仁、山茱萸、熟地黄、菟丝子、狗脊等。

养心、肝、脾、肺、肾常用的食物：动物的肉、心、肝、肚、肾、鞭、脑髓、肺等。

养筋、骨、肤、发、齿常用的中药：杜仲、补骨脂、鹿角、鹿茸、菟丝子、肉苁蓉、续断、五加皮、何首乌、核桃仁、大枣、怀山药、莲子、黑芝麻、桑椹、枸杞子等。

养筋、骨、肤、发、齿常用的食物：动物的骨、肾、筋、肉、尾，牛肉，燕窝，蛋，冰糖，蜜糖，花生等。

药膳的种类及制作方法有哪些？

中国传统药膳的制作和应用，不但是一门科学，更可以说是一门艺术。药膳的形式繁多，大体有汤、羹、粥、糊、饼、卷、锅贴、包子、冻、汤丸、糕等，其基本制作方法有蒸、煎、煮、炖、煲、焖、煨、烧、炒、炸、烤等。

药膳的分类有哪些？

大致来说，按照药膳的功用，可分为滋阴类、壮阳类、益气类、补血类、养心安神类、补肺类、滋肝明目类、补肾益精类、健脾开胃类、强筋壮骨类、润肤泽容类、调和五脏类、乌发固齿类等。

滋阴类药膳常用的药物和食物有哪些？具有什么功效？

滋阴类药膳选用滋阴药物，配合食物烹调制成。

滋阴类药膳常选用的中药有生地黄、黄精、桑椹、女贞子、枸杞子、玄参、熟地黄、天冬、麦冬、沙参、玉竹。选用的食物主要有甲鱼、乌龟、燕窝、银耳、海参。

滋阴类药膳的功效为养阴增液，生津止渴，清热除烦。适用于素体阴液不足，或久病耗阴所致的肢体羸瘦、面容憔悴、口燥咽干、虚烦不眠，甚则骨蒸盗汗、呛咳无痰，颧部发红，梦遗滑精，腰酸背痛。

滋阴类药膳多甘寒滋腻，凡脾胃虚弱，痰湿内阻，腹满便溏及适逢外感者，均不宜用。

滋阴类药膳举隅

生地黄鸡 （《饮膳正要》）

组成： 生地黄 250g，饴糖 150g，乌鸡 1 只。

制作方法： 上三味，将乌鸡宰杀后，除去毛桩和内脏，冲洗干净；生地黄切成细丝，与饴糖拌匀，放入鸡腹内。将鸡装入盆内，加清水适量。置蒸笼中，用武火蒸至熟透即成。

功效： 滋阴补肾。适用于腰背疼痛，骨髓虚损，不能久立，身重气乏，盗汗少食，时复吐利。

黄精炖猪瘦肉 （民间方）

组成： 黄精 50g，猪瘦肉 200g，葱、生姜、食盐、料酒各适量。

制作方法： 将黄精、猪瘦肉洗净，分别切成长 3cm、宽 1.5cm 的条块，放入瓦锅（砂锅）内，加水适量，放入葱、生姜、食盐、料酒，隔水炖煮。

功效： 养脾阴，益心肺。适用于阴虚体质的平时调养，以及心脾阴血不足所致的食少、失眠等症。

桑椹醪（《食鉴本草》）

　　组成： 鲜桑椹 1000g，糯米 500g，酒曲适量。

　　制作方法： 将鲜桑椹洗净捣汁（或以干品 300g 煎汁去渣），再将药汁与糯米共同烧煮，做成糯米干饭，待冷加酒曲适量拌匀，发酵成酒酿，每日随量佐餐食用。

　　功效： 补血益肾，聪耳明目。适用于肝肾阴亏消渴、便秘、耳鸣、目暗、瘰疬、关节不利等症。

壮阳类药膳常用的药物和食物有哪些？有什么功效？

　　壮阳类药膳选用温热壮阳中药配合一定食物烹调而成。

　　壮阳类药膳常选用的中药有鹿角、干姜，以及牛鞭、动物肾等。选用的食物有羊肉、鹿肉等。

　　壮阳类药膳的功效为壮阳补肾，温里散寒，益精补血。适用于阳痿、遗精、白浊、带下、腰膝酸软、畏寒肢冷、食少腹泻等症。

　　壮阳类药膳温热而燥，凡热性病，阴虚内热、痈疽疮毒者等均不能食用，此类药膳以冬季食用为佳。

壮阳类药膳举隅

鹿角粥（《臞仙活人方》）

　　组成： 鹿角粉 5 ~ 10g，粳米 30 ~ 60g，食盐少许。

　　制作方法： 先以粳米煮粥，米汤煮沸后调入鹿角粉，加入少许食盐，同煮为粥，一日分两次服。

　　功效： 补肾阳，益精血，强筋骨。适用于肾阳不足，精血亏虚之畏寒身冷，腰膝酸痛，阳痿早泄，不孕不育，精神疲乏；小儿发育不良，骨软行迟，囟门不合；妇女崩漏、带下；阴疽内陷，疮疡久溃不敛等。宜冬季服食。素体有热，阴虚阳亢，或阳虚外感发热者均不宜食用。

益气类药膳常用的药物和食物有哪些？有什么功效？

　　益气类药膳选用益气中药配用补脾健胃食物烹制而成。

　　益气类药膳常选用的中药有人参、党参、黄芪、怀山药等。选用的食物有鸡、鱼、猪肉等。

益气类药膳的功效为益气补中，健运脾胃。适用于肺脾气虚的短气咳喘、乏力神疲、食少纳差，以及年老体弱、久病脱肛等症。

此类药膳为补益之品，不宜一次食用太多，宜少量久食；身体羸弱之人更须防虚不胜补。凡实证、热证、外感病症初期等不可服用。

益气类药膳举隅

清蒸参芪鸡 （《常见慢性病食物疗养法》）

组成： 党参 30g，蜜炙黄芪 60g，母鸡一只（1000～1500g），细盐、黄酒适量。

制作方法： 党参切片冲洗净后，用黄酒一匙浸润。母鸡杀后去毛，剖腹洗净，切成小块。将鸡块、党参、蜜炙黄芪放碗内，撒上细盐一匙，淋上黄酒一匙，蒸 3 小时至鸡肉熟烂即可。分 2～3 天吃完。

功效： 补气益胃，补虚固脱。适用于身体虚弱、畏冷，年老气虚脱肛，多食易饥等症。

牛乳粥 （《养生与长寿》）

组成： 牛乳 500ml，大米适量。

制作方法： 将大米淘洗净下锅煮，至半熟时加入牛乳同煮熟即可。

功效： 益气补虚。适用于脾胃气虚、身体虚弱等症。

补血类药膳常用的药物和食物有哪些？有什么功效？

补血类药膳选用具有补血功效的中药与食物配合，经烹调而成。

补血类药膳常用的中药有当归、熟地黄、党参、黄芪、阿胶、白芍、川芎、田七、枸杞子、鸡血藤。选用的食物主要有羊肉、牛肉、鸡、鸭等。

补血类药膳的功效为补血养血，适用于血虚所致的面色无华，神疲乏力，头昏眼花、心悸失眠、月经失调等症。

此类药膳多属滑腻之品，故实热、痰湿中满、外感发热者不可食用。

补血类药膳举隅

田七炖鸡 （《养生食疗菜谱》）

组成： 母鸡肉 1300g，田七 15g，姜块 20g，葱 30g，精盐 10g，绍酒 30g。

制作方法：将田七制成粉末，母鸡肉、姜块、葱洗净。砂锅加清水，放入鸡肉，旺火烧开后，撇去血沫，加姜块、葱、绍酒，转小火炖至软烂，加田七粉、精盐，调味即成。

功效：补血益气，活血散瘀。适用于妇女产后气血不足，小腹疼痛，恶露不尽及肺痨咳血等病症。

阿胶白皮粥 （《养生食疗菜谱》）

组成：阿胶 15g，桑白皮 15g，糯米 100g，红糖 8g。

制作方法：将桑白皮洗净，放入砂锅煎汁，取汁两次。再将糯米淘洗干净，放入锅中，加清水煮 10 分钟后，倒入药汁、阿胶，再放入红糖，煮成粥。

功效：滋阴补血，润燥清肺。适用于阴血亏虚，肺阴亏耗、津伤液燥所致久咳、咯血、便血、月经过少、崩漏、胎动不安等症。

第五节
进食宜忌

进食食量多少为宜？

《黄帝内经》中强调"饮食有节"，主要是指饮食应该定时定量，食不过饱是古代饮食养生的首要原则。因为"饮食自倍，脾胃乃伤"，饱食是脾胃受损的一个重要原因。隋代《诸病源候论》指出，过饱除了引起烦闷、睡眠不好之外，还容易引起积聚不消，上腹部包块疼痛、四肢关节不利、面部发黑生斑、腰痛、水肿，重者可能百脉闭阻，以致减损寿命。饮食量因人而异，《备急千金要方》认为正确的方法是"言语既慎，仍节饮食。是以善养性者，先饥而食，先渴而饮；食欲数而少，不欲顿而多，则难消也。常欲令如饱中饥，饥中饱耳。盖饱则伤肺，饥则伤气……故每学淡食，食当熟嚼，使米脂入腹，勿使酒脂入肠"。强调饮食要有节制、有规律性，建议少吃多餐，不能一次吃得太多，否则难以消化。要经常保持那种饱而不胀满，饿而不虚空的状态。宋代名士苏东坡有"三养"名言："安分以养福，宽胃以养气，省责以养财。"其中"安分"与"省责"是处世的经验，而"宽胃"就是要使肠胃处于一种宽舒通畅的状态，不能把胃塞得太满了。

古人对进食时间有何建议？

古人的一日三餐，对晚饭的戒律最多，唐末《医心方》中专设了一篇"夜食禁"，提出"夜食恒不欲满，令人无病"，如果夜食过饱又不活动，则不易消化而导致疾病。清代石成金提出了晚饭最佳时间："大约午饭宜在午前，而晚饭宜在日未落时。总之饭后宜多过一时，使饮食稍下方睡，则无患矣。"古人认为在七点以后吃晚饭就是不合适的了。

古人对进食速度有何建议？

《老老恒言》引华佗《食论》曰："食物有三化：一火化，烂煮也；一口化，细嚼也；一腹化，入胃自化也。"就是说进食宜细嚼慢咽，进食速度不宜过快，尤其是对于肠胃不好者及老年人来说，消化食物靠肠胃本身已经负担很重了，因此，把食物煮烂及细嚼慢咽是帮助消化的好办法。清代医家石成金列举了细嚼慢咽的三大好处："盖细嚼则食之精华能滋补五脏，一也；脾胃易于消化，二也；不至吞呛噎咳，三也。"

古人对饮食口味有何建议？

古人主张饮食宜淡，这里"淡"有两层含义：一是素淡，与食物品类的肥甘醇厚相对应；一是味淡，与味道之咸相对应。关于饮食素淡，古人的论述比较多，从《素问》开始，古人就崇尚素淡饮食，而对过食肥腻厚味的大鱼大肉持批评态度。《素问》认为正常人过食"膏粱厚味"，即过食肥腻、味道厚重的食物，足以引起疮疡类疾病。而患者更应注意饮食素淡，如"病热少愈，食肉则复，多食则遗"，就是说，得热性病到了快痊愈的时候，吃了肉就会复发，甚至稍多进食也会引起一些后遗症。后世医家多继承此观点，如唐代孙思邈《备急千金要方》中载"每食不用重肉，喜生百病"。古代主张多吃味淡之食的言论出现得比较晚，明确的论述可见于清代《长生秘诀》："淡食最补人，五味各有所伤……五味中，而咸味又能凝血滞气，伤人更甚。"认为过食咸味可以使面色枯槁，血脉壅塞。

古代饮食禁忌有哪些？

饮食禁忌也称"食禁"，或"食忌"。古代的饮食禁忌内容比较广泛，包括有毒物品的禁忌、各类特殊人群的饮食禁忌、各种食物相互搭配的禁忌、患者及服药期间的饮食禁忌等。最早入载于《汉书·艺文志》的是《神农黄帝食禁》。隋唐以前，有许多关于饮食禁忌的书，如《老子禁食经》《神农食忌》《扁鹊食禁》等。

有毒物品是早期饮食保健最为重视的问题。这些物品本身具有毒性，有的是由于污染，或久置腐烂，或因其他因素而产生毒性。被后世人尊为医圣的汉代名医张仲景，在他的著作中，就附有"禽兽虫鱼禁忌并治""果实菜谷禁忌并治"，总结了汉以前的动、植物类食物的禁忌，并列举了许多食物中毒的解救方法。

古代有关动物的食用禁忌很多，在《养生食忌》中，这种禁忌甚至泛滥到凡是形态怪异、与众不同的动物和植物，都被认为对人体不利。例如：爪子长得特别大的不能吃，鱼类的鱼鳞或鱼鳃逆生的不能吃、鱼目能开合的不能吃。

特殊人群的禁忌，俗称"忌口"。所谓特殊人群，较受重视的是小儿、孕产期妇女、老人及患者。中医对各类特殊人群的饮食是十分注意的，服药的患者更应注意不得进食与所服药物性质相反或不利于药物发挥作用的食物。唐代《食疗本草》中记载"小儿不得与炒豆食之，若食了，忽食猪肉，必壅气致死，十有八九"。小儿脾胃功能尚未健全，豆类食物本就难以消化，炒豆更甚，这时如再吃油腻的猪肉，虽说不至于"十死八九"，但自然是不利于小儿健康的。古代最为讲究的是孕产期妇女的饮食禁忌。总的原则是"产前宜凉，产后宜温"。因为产前多食热性食物，容易引起胎动不安，且可能使婴儿易患疮疡疖肿类疾病；产后恶露未净，如果多食寒凉性食物，就会使瘀血停留，引起恶露不尽、产后腹痛等。哺乳期妇女，同样要注意饮食，有些食物可能使乳汁减少，像酸石榴。还有些食物可能通过乳汁进入婴儿体内，引起婴儿的相应不良反应，俗称"过奶"。

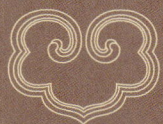

第六章

药　养

第一节
药养概述

何谓药养?

中药养生是在中医理论指导下，通过内服或外用中药并借助其补养或通泻作用，对机体进行综合调整，调和气血、平衡阴阳、和调脏腑、畅通经络，以达增进健康、延年益寿的养生方法。

药养的特点有哪些?

《黄帝内经》中就提出了"治未病"的预防思想，《素问·四气调神大论》曰："是故圣人不治已病治未病，不治已乱治未乱，此之谓也。夫病已成而后药之，乱已成而后治之，譬犹渴而穿井，斗而铸锥，不亦晚乎?"非常生动地说明了治未病的意义，并进一步阐释了药物养生在疾病预防和治疗中的重要作用。概括之，药物养生具有以下三个特点。

第一，未病先防。疾病的发生关系到正邪两个方面，药物养生的作用也是在正邪两个方面共同作用。首先是调养身体，提高正气抗邪能力。《素问遗篇·刺法论》云："正气存内，邪不可干。"对于体质虚弱，正气不足者，适当服用补益药物可扶助正气，增强体质，防止疾病的发生。其次是避其毒气，防止病邪的侵害。《素问·上古天真论》曰："虚邪贼风，避之有时。"药物养生除提高正气，增强抗病能力外，还可防止病邪的侵害。如用贯众、板蓝根、大青叶等预防流感，用茵陈、栀子等预防肝炎，用马齿苋等预防菌痢等，均收到很好的防治效果。

第二，既病防变。如果疾病已发生，则应争取早期诊断、早期治疗，以药物调养防止疾病发展和传变。《素问·阴阳应象大论》云："邪风之至，疾如风雨，故善治者治皮毛，其次治肌肤，其次治筋脉，其次治六腑，其次治五脏。治五脏者，半生半死也。"说明外邪侵入人体，如不及时诊治，病邪会由表及里，步步深入，加重病情，因此要尽早治疗，以防疾病入里，侵犯五脏，使病情复杂深重。《难经·七十七难》云："上工治未病，中工治已病……所谓治未病者，见肝之病，则知肝当传之于脾，故先实其脾气，无令得受肝之邪。故曰治未病焉。中工者，见肝之病，不晓相传，但一心治肝，故曰治已病也。"这是既病防变法则的具体应用，根据既病传变规律，先安未受邪之地，防止疾病的传变、蔓延，以保护未病脏腑。

第三，瘥后防复。病后应该用适当的药物调养，使机体正气恢复，气血流畅，脏腑得养，阴平阳秘，不再受邪而复发。如《伤寒论》云："伤寒解后，虚赢少气，气逆欲呕，竹叶石膏汤主之。"意思是外感热病缓解后，身体赢瘦，气短乏力，午后低热，此为残热未尽，虚热上扰所致，治宜竹叶石膏汤，益气生津，甘寒清热，使余邪得清，气阴得养。

药养的原理是什么？

人体健康长寿很重要的条件是先天禀赋强盛，后天营养充足。此外，还需阴阳平衡、气血调和、经脉畅通。肾为先天之本，脾胃为后天之本，因此药物养生多立足于固护先天、后天，以脾肾为重点，兼顾五脏、气血、阴阳等，通过培补先天、调理脾胃、协调五脏、平衡阴阳、调和气血、畅通经络，而达到补养身体，益寿延年，祛病强身的功效。

第二节
古代药养常用中药

具有养生保健作用的中药有多少？

中医四大经典之一的《神农本草经》中说："上药一百二十种为君，主养命以应天。""中药一百二十种为臣，主养性以应人。""下药一百二十五种为佐使，主治病以应地。"在《神农本草经》365种药物中，记述有延年、不老、耐老、益气、轻身、增寿等作用的药物有165种。明代李时珍的《本草纲目》记载1892种药物，具有抗衰老、延年作用的药物有253种，并选录延寿方剂89首。清代宫廷热衷于服用长生不老方药，因此宫中此类医方甚多，如益寿膏、补益资生丸、菊花延龄膏、百龄丸、松龄太平春酒等。

古代常用养身益寿中药有哪些？

古代常用的养身益寿中药有人参、鹿茸、冬虫夏草、阿胶、枸杞子、熟地黄、生地黄、肉苁蓉、巴戟天、菟丝子、茯苓、牛膝、天冬、远志、杜仲、五味子、白术、菖蒲、当归、麦冬、山茱萸、何首乌、补骨脂、山药、黄芪、薏苡仁、龙眼肉、玉竹、黄精、桑椹、女贞子、刺五加、党参、酸枣仁、甘草、大枣等。其中以补肾填精药使用频率最高，其次为健脾益气药和养心安神药。

补气类中药有哪些？

补气类中药具有强壮作用，能增强体力，主要适用于气虚证，尤其是肺脾气虚。补气类常见药物介绍如下。

人参

为五加科植物人参的根及根茎。性微温，味甘、微苦。归脾、肺经。具有大补元气、生津止渴、益智安神之功效。其所含的主要成分有人参皂苷、氨基酸等。可用于治疗体弱乏力、口渴喜饮、多梦眠差、自汗、怔忡、呕吐不食、胃脘冷痛、气短久咳、性欲减退等症状。

人参的品类有很多，因加工方法及野生与栽培的不同，分为野山参、移山参、园参、生晒参、红参、白参等。野生者称为野山参；将野山参的幼苗从野外移植后经过人工培植者称为移山参；人工培植者称为园参；直接晒干者称为生晒参；蒸熟后晒干者称为红参（大力参）；煮后再入糖汁中浸后晒干者，为白参。其中野山参以年代久远者为佳，补力较大；人工培植的园参，补力较弱。红参比生晒参作用效力强，白参较弱。人参自古至今一直被视为珍贵的补品，但人参终归是药物，不可滥用，过量服用人参可引起便秘、鼻衄、腹胀、失眠、烦躁等症状，使用时应当注意。

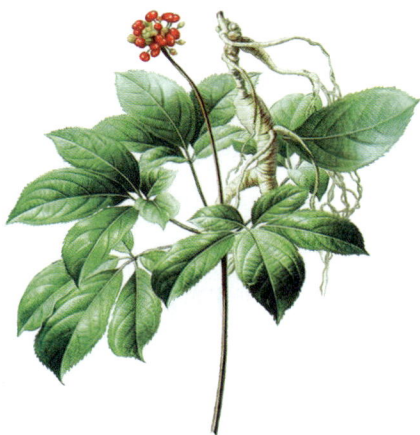

人参

黄芪

为豆科植物膜荚黄芪或蒙古黄芪的根。性温，味甘，归脾、肺经。有补气升阳，固表止汗，托疮生肌，利尿消肿之功效。黄芪蜜炙，补气力量增强，用于补气时，宜用蜜炙黄芪；用于止汗、利水、托疮生肌时，宜用生黄芪。可用于治疗体弱乏力、自汗盗汗、血虚头晕、慢性肝炎、肢麻身痛、浮肿尿少、痈疽不溃等病症。

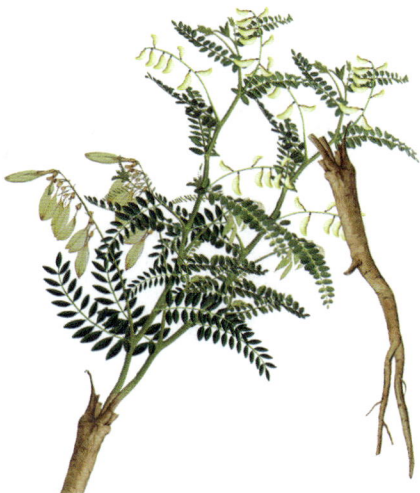

黄芪

白术

为菊科植物白术的根茎。性温，味甘、苦，归脾、胃经。有补脾益气、燥湿利水、固表止汗的功效，为补脾燥湿要药。健脾和胃宜用焦白术或炒白术；健脾止泻时宜用土炒白术；利水消肿、固表止汗时宜用生白术。可用于治疗腹胀纳差、脾虚泄泻、自汗盗汗、伤暑泄泻、痰饮水肿、小儿流涎等病症。

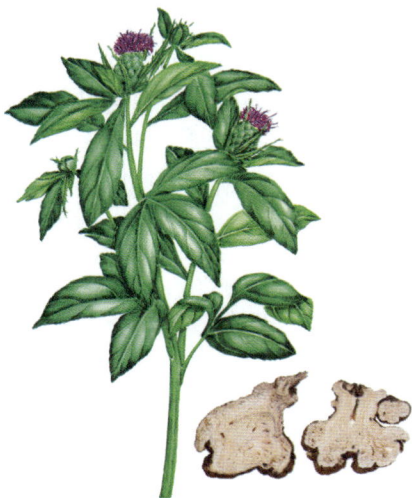

白术

补血类中药有哪些？

补血类中药主要用于血虚证。血虚证的表现有：面色无华、唇甲苍白、眩晕心悸、女子月经不调等。补血类常见药物介绍如下。

当归

为伞形科植物当归的根。性温，味甘、辛、苦，归心、肝、肺、脾经。具有补血调经、活血止痛、润肠通便的功效，为治疗血证之要品。补血宜用当归身，活血宜用当归尾，和血宜用全当归；补血润肠宜用生当归，通经活血宜用炒当归（酒炒）。可用于治疗气血两虚证、虚寒腹痛、血虚便秘、月经不调、产后腹痛、慢性肝炎、慢性气管炎等病症。凡湿盛中满、大便泄泻、经多崩漏者，不宜使用。

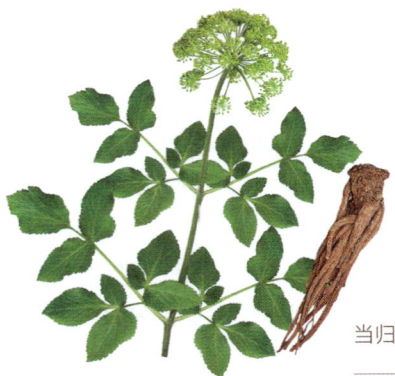

当归

阿胶

为马科动物驴的皮，经漂泡去毛后熬制而成的胶块。原药打碎用，或用蛤粉、蒲黄粉炒成阿胶珠用（清肺宜蛤粉炒、止血宜蒲黄炒）。性平，味甘，归肝、肺、肾经。具有补血止血、滋阴润燥的功效。单用或配伍应用可用于冬季进补（阿胶、黄酒、核桃仁、黑芝麻、红枣、龙眼肉等），还可用于治疗眩晕心悸、心烦失眠、久咳燥咳、吐血衄血、经多崩漏等病症。阿胶甘平质黏，为血肉有情之品，为治血虚的要药。本品用于止血时，需注意病证属实热或夹有瘀滞者，不宜用之过早，否则有留瘀之弊。生阿胶容易碍胃，脾胃功能虚弱的人群应用时应当注意。

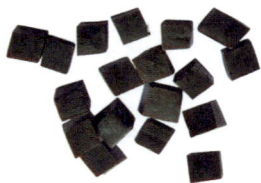

阿胶

熟地黄

为生地黄的加工品。性微温，味甘，归心、肝、肾经。具有补血调经，滋肾育阴的功效。可治疗气血虚弱、精血不足等引起的

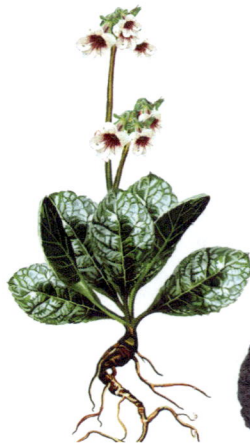

熟地黄

病症。熟地黄不仅滋阴养血，还可生精补髓壮骨，为补益肝肾之常用药。熟地黄性质黏腻，有碍脾胃运化，凡脾胃虚弱、气滞痰多、腹满便溏者，用药时宜注意。临证处方时，为防止其滋腻碍胃之弊，常配伍砂仁使用，或与芳香健胃药同用。

补阴类中药有哪些?

补阴类中药具有养阴、增液、润燥的作用，适用于阴虚液亏诸证。补阴类常见药物介绍如下。

北沙参

为伞形科植物珊瑚菜的根。性微寒，味甘、微苦，归肺、胃经。具有润肺止咳、益胃生津的功效。可治疗口渴舌干、劳嗽痰血、阴虚燥咳等病症。不宜用于虚寒之证。

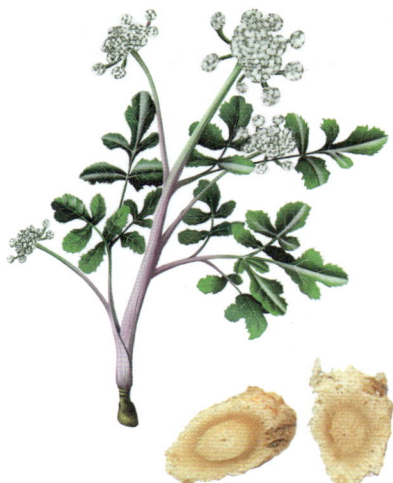

北沙参

石斛

为兰科植物金钗石斛或其多种同属植物的茎。性寒，味甘，归肺、胃、肾经。具有养胃生津、滋阴除热的功效，为滋养胃阴的常用药。可治疗舌干口渴、长期低热、干咳无痰、视力减退等病症。

龟甲

为龟科动物乌龟的背甲及腹甲。性平，味甘、咸，归肾、心、肝经。具有滋阴潜阳、益肾强骨、固精止崩的功效。可治疗惊悸失眠、头晕目眩、经多崩漏、筋骨不健等病症。本品为咸寒之物，故脾胃虚寒、外感邪气未解者不宜使用。

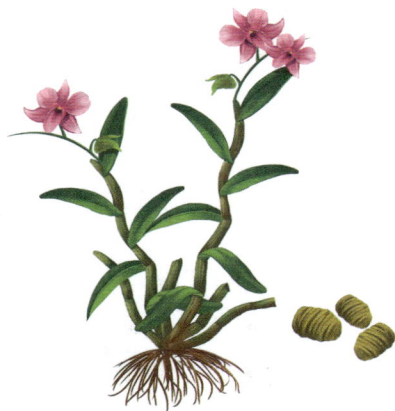

石斛

补阳类中药有哪些?

补阳类中药主要用于阳虚证。阳虚证包括心阳虚、脾阳虚、肾阳虚等证，因肾为先天之本，故补阳常从补肾阳入手。补阳类中药一般具有温肾壮阳、补精髓、强筋骨等作用。补阳类常见药物介绍如下。

鹿茸

为鹿科动物梅花鹿或马鹿的雄鹿头上未骨化而带毛茸的幼角。鹿茸成长至茸毛脱落，硬化为骨质者为鹿角，鹿角熬成胶者，为鹿角胶。熬膏剩余的骨渣，为鹿角霜。性温，味甘、咸，归肝、肾经。具有补肾阳、益精血、强筋骨的功效。可用于治疗身体虚弱、心脏衰弱、肾亏精虚、小儿发育不良、带下、崩漏、贫血等病症。

鹿茸与肉桂、附子等药都有补阳作用，但桂、附性热刚燥，适用于真阳衰微，而不宜用于精髓不足；鹿茸为血肉有情之品，甘温质柔，补阳兼生精，既可用于真阳不足，也可用于精髓亏虚。

冬虫夏草

为麦角菌科真菌冬虫夏草寄生在蝙蝠蛾科昆虫幼虫上的子座和幼虫尸体的复合体。性温，味甘，归肺、肾经。具有滋肺补肾、止血化痰的功效。可用于体弱多病者的补益，治疗肺结核、慢性肾炎、阳痿遗精等病症。冬虫夏草既能滋肺，又能补肾阳，凡阴虚阳浮而为虚喘或咳嗽痰血之证，用之甚效。近年来常用作调补之品，有表证及肺热咳血者忌用。

巴戟天

为茜草科植物巴戟天的根。性微温，味辛、甘，归肾、肝经。具有补肾壮阳、强筋骨、逐寒湿的功效。可治疗小便频数、肾虚阳痿、风湿痹痛、经寒腹痛等病症。巴戟天为助阳之品，适用于虚寒证，凡阴虚火旺、口干舌燥、大便燥结者忌用。

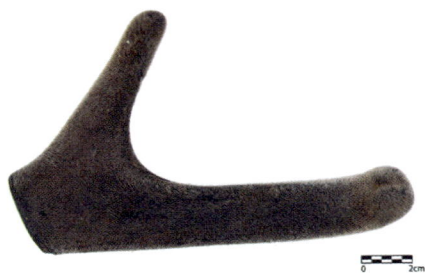

鹿茸

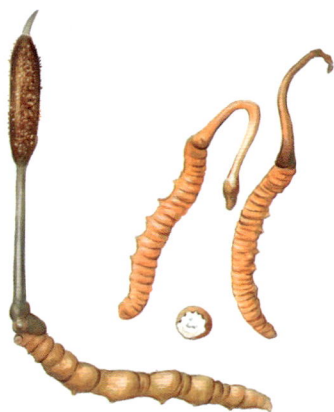

冬虫夏草

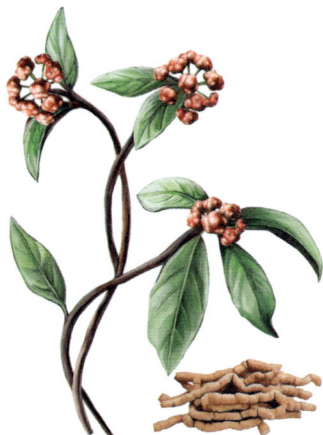

巴戟天

第三节
养身益寿常用名方

养身益寿方剂的组方原则是什么？

养身益寿方剂多为年老体弱者而设，故补益之法成为主要治法。其方剂组成原则主要如下。

第一，动静结合。养身益寿方剂多为补益之品，其性壅滞黏腻，守而不走，即药之"静"者。而补益药物需达病所方能起到效用，因此需借气血之循行方可布散，故需行气、活血等药之"动"者，动静结合，亦养亦行，相得益彰，共同发挥补益功效。

第二，补泻结合。补泻结合是方剂组方配伍原则之一。通过药物的补与泻，共奏阴平阳秘、气血平衡之功效。临床常见的补肾阴名方六味地黄丸，它的组方特点就是补中有泻，三补三泻，平补平泻。其中三补指的是山茱萸、熟地黄和山药，其中熟地黄滋阴补肾，山茱萸滋肾益肝，而山药可以肝、脾、肾同补。三泻指的是方中的牡丹皮、茯苓、泽泻，可以帮助泻肝火、渗湿降浊，防止滋补之品太过于滋腻，不利于药物的吸收，诸药配伍，共奏补益肝肾之功。

第三，寒热平调。药性有寒、热、温、凉之别。使用药物，不宜过偏，过寒伤阳，过热伤阴，故组方时多寒热配伍使用，使寒而无过，热而不燥，寒热适中。如韩懋治疗失眠的名方交泰丸中，黄连配伍肉桂，一寒一热，寒热并用，相辅相成，交通心肾，使水火既济，对心肾不交的失眠有良好的治疗作用。

第四，相辅相成。养身益寿方剂的组方立足于辨证，着眼于整体，方剂中各味药物有机配合，既突出其主治功效，又兼顾旁证、兼证，主次分明，结构严谨，相互搭配，相辅相成。方剂中开、阖、补、泻合用，升、降、通、塞并用，寒热并用，此即为相辅相成共同起效。

养身益寿方剂的功效和应用范围是什么？

养身益寿方剂组成多为补益药物，为针对虚证而设，概括而言，功效有三个方面：一是提高机体抵抗力，增强免疫能力；二是补虚治病，调节和改善人体生理功能；三是抗衰老、益寿延年。适用于先天不足，体质虚弱、病后及产后体虚，中老年体虚，肿瘤辅助治疗等，还可用于养生防病、益寿延年。

养身益寿方剂的常用剂型有哪些？

古人认为："汤者荡也，去大病用之。散者散也，去急病用之。丸者缓也，不能速去之。"养身益寿方剂常用的剂型有汤剂（煎剂）、散剂、丸剂、膏剂、丹剂等。此外，还有药酒、药膳、药茶等。

汤剂，是将一味或多味药物加水浸泡煎煮，去渣取汁的液体制剂，一般作内服用。特点是吸收快、作用迅速。

散剂，是将药物粉碎、均匀混合成的粉末状制剂，可内服，可外用。特点是制作简便、节省药材、不易变质。

丸剂，可分为蜜丸、水丸、糊丸、浓缩丸等。是将药物研成细末，用蜜、水、米糊、面糊或药汁等作为赋形剂制成的球形固体制剂。特点是体积小、易贮存、药力持久、吸收缓慢。

膏剂，一般指煎膏剂，又称为膏滋或膏方，是将药材反复煎煮到一定程度后去渣取汁浓缩，再加入适当的辅料制成的半流体制剂。膏方是中国江南地区常用的冬令进补方式，其优点是口感滑润爽口，既能进补，又能防病治病。

丹剂，因主要由精炼药品或贵重药品制成，故不称丸剂而称丹剂。有些剂量小、作用大的散剂也称作丹。部分外科使用的丹剂，指含有汞、硫黄等矿物，经过加热升华提炼而成的一种制剂，具有剂量小、作用大、含矿物质的特点，如红升丹、白降丹等。此外，习惯上把某些较贵重的药品或有特殊功效的药物剂型叫作丹，如至宝丹、紫雪丹等。所以，丹剂并非一种固定的剂型。

药酒，是将中药材浸泡在白酒或黄酒中，经过一段时间后，中药材中的有效成分溶解在酒中，经过滤去渣后得到的澄明液体制剂，可供内服或外用。药酒具有配制方便、药性稳定、安全有效的特点。由于酒精是一种良好的半极性有机溶剂，中药的各种有效成分易溶于其中，药借酒力、酒助药势而充分发挥其效力，提高疗效。从古传至今的著名药酒有御酒堂，现在新兴的药酒有龟寿酒、劲酒等。中医理论认为慢性虚损性疾病日久必将导致正气亏虚、脉络瘀阻。药酒配方具有补血益气、滋阴温阳的作用，同时酒本身又有辛散温通的功效。因此药酒可广泛应用于各种慢性虚损性疾病的防治，并能抗衰老、延年益寿。

药膳，是药物与食物结合，经过烹饪加工制成的一种具有食疗作用的膳食。它是中国传统的医学知识与烹调经验相结合的产物。它"寓医于食"，既将药物作为食物，又将食物赋以药用，药借食力，食助药威，是一种兼有药物功效和食品美味的特殊膳食，既具有营养价值，又可防病治病、保健强身、延年益寿。

药茶，也称中药代茶饮，指以中草药与茶叶配用，或以中草药（单味或复方）或者药物粗粉代茶冲泡、煎煮，像茶一样饮用的制剂。中药代茶饮为中国的传统剂型，是在中医理、法、方、药理论指导下，依据辨证或辨证与辨病相结合，为防治疾病、病后调理或养生保健而形成的剂型。具有调配方便、针对性强、灵活度大等特点，十分适宜于疾病调治与养生康复。它既保持了中医汤剂辨证论治加减灵活、疗效显著的特色，又克服了煎煮烦琐、携带不方便等缺点，与现代生活节奏加快的发展趋势相适应。

养身益寿方剂有哪些分类？

人体虚损不足的类型有很多，养身益寿方剂中药的作用重点也有不同，按照补益虚损的作用不同，养身益寿方剂可分为养心类、养肝类、养脾类、养肺类、养肾类和养五脏类。此外，还有美容养颜类方剂和健脑益智类方剂。

养心类名方举隅

神仙保精延驻饵茯苓方 （出自《太平圣惠方》）

组成： 茯苓、松脂、钟乳粉、白蜜。
功用： 补心肾，益精神。
主治： 心肾不足，失眠健忘，神衰乏力。

四补丸 （出自《圣济总录》）

组成： 柏子仁、何首乌、肉苁蓉、牛膝。
功用： 补肾，养心，安神。
主治： 肾虚，心神不宁，失眠健忘，腰膝无力。

定志补心汤 （出自《千金翼方》）

组成： 远志、菖蒲、人参、茯苓。
功用： 补心气。
主治： 心气不足，心痛惊恐。

养心延龄益寿丹 （出自《慈禧太后医方选议》）

组成： 茯神、当归、酒白芍、牡丹皮、干地黄、炒枳壳、酸枣仁、丹参、柏子仁、川芎、炒于术、陈皮、酒条芩、栀子。
功用： 养心安神，养血柔肝。
主治： 肝火郁热，心神失养，体瘦气怯，神虚不易安眠，咽干，足心热。

养肝类名方举隅

明目益肾丸 （出自《丹溪心法》）

组成： 枸杞子、当归、生地黄、茯神、菟丝子、知母、黄柏、山药、巴戟天、五味子、天冬、人参、菊花。

功用： 滋阴补肾，清养肝目。

主治： 肝肾虚，相火旺，气阴不足，眩晕目糊。

明目延龄膏 （出自《慈禧太后医方选议》）

组成： 桑叶、菊花。

功用： 柔肝明目。

主治： 肝火偏旺，头晕眼花。

神仙驻颜延年方 （出自《普济方》）

组成： 枳实、熟地黄、菊花、天冬。

功用： 养肝肾，明目。

主治： 肝肾不足，视物模糊，心下痞满。

杞菊地黄丸 （出自《医级》）

组成： 枸杞子、菊花、熟地黄、山茱萸、山药、茯苓、泽泻、牡丹皮。

功用： 补肾，养肝，明目。

主治： 肝肾虚，头晕眼花，消渴。

养脾类名方举隅

守中丸 （出自《圣济总录》）

组成： 生地黄、人参、白术、甘菊花、山药、枸杞子、茯苓、麦冬。

功用： 补气健脾，益肾养肝。

主治： 后天不足，先天失养，头晕目眩，腰胁不适，形体消瘦。

健脾汤 （出自《千金翼方》）

组成： 生地黄、黄芪、芍药、甘草、生姜、白蜜。

功用： 养阴血，健脾胃。

主治： 气血不调，人重如磐石，欲食即呕，四肢酸削不收。

扶元和中膏 （出自《慈禧太后医方选议》）

组成： 党参、白术、茯苓、当归身、杜仲、生黄芪、炒谷芽、鸡内金、砂仁、佩兰、香附、生姜、姜半夏、大枣。

功用： 扶元和中。

主治： 久病脾虚食少，胸闷干呕，倒饱嘈杂，食物不消。

木香人参散 （出自《寿亲养老新书》）

组成： 木香、人参、白术、丁香、炙甘草、厚朴、干姜、陈皮、茯苓、肉豆蔻、枇杷叶、藿香叶。

功用： 温中理气。

主治： 老人脾胃虚寒，脘腹胀痛，痰逆呕恶，大便失调。

养肺类名方举隅

琼玉膏 （出自《丹溪心法》）

组成： 人参、茯苓、生地黄、白蜜。

功用： 益气阴，养心肺。

主治： 虚劳咳嗽，短气无力。

补肺散 （出自《千金翼方》）

组成： 白石英、五味子、桂心、大枣、麦冬、款冬花、桑白皮、干姜、甘草。

功用： 温心肾，补肺气。

主治： 肺气不足，胸痛牵背，上气失声。

养肾类名方举隅

菟丝子丸 （出自《济生方》）

组成： 菟丝子、杜仲、熟地黄、鹿茸、肉苁蓉、车前子、桂心、牛膝、附子。

功用： 温补肾阳。

主治： 腰膝酸冷，四肢不温，男子阳事不举，女子宫寒不孕等。

大补阴丸 （出自《丹溪心法》）

组成： 炒黄柏、炒知母、熟地黄、龟甲。

功用： 滋阴降火。

主治： 阴虚火旺，潮热盗汗，痿弱无力。

二至丸 （出自《普济方》）

组成： 女贞子、墨旱莲。

功用： 滋阴养血。

主治： 阴虚，肝肾不足，眩晕，失眠，腰膝酸软，须发早白。

延寿丹 （出自《世补斋医书》）

组成： 何首乌、豨莶草、菟丝子、杜仲、牛膝、女贞子、桑叶、忍冬藤、生地黄、桑椹膏、黑芝麻膏、金樱子膏、墨旱莲膏。

功用： 滋肾养肝，强筋骨，祛风。

主治： 肝肾虚，阴血衰，眩晕腰酸，发白早衰。

益寿养真膏 （出自《东医宝鉴》）

组成： 生地黄、人参、茯苓、天冬、麦冬、地骨皮、蜜。

功用： 益气养阴，填精补髓。

主治： 诸虚百损，瘫痪，劳瘵，五脏不足，精神不振。

养五脏类名方举隅

养寿丹 （出自《御药院方》）

组成： 远志、菖蒲、巴戟天、白术、茯苓、地骨皮、续断、枸杞子、菊花、细辛、地黄、车前子、何首乌、牛膝、肉苁蓉、菟丝子、覆盆子。

功用： 补养五脏。

主治： 五脏虚损，麻痛，须发早白，筋骨无力。

斑龙二至百补丸 （出自《景岳全书》）

组成： 鹿角、黄精、枸杞子、熟地黄、菟丝子、金樱子、天冬、麦冬、牛膝、楮实子、龙眼肉、鹿角霜、人参、黄芪、芡实、茯苓、山药、山茱萸、生地黄、知母、五味子。

功用： 固本保元，调理五脏。

主治： 五脏虚损，骨蒸羸瘦，或不育。

美容养颜类名方举隅

七白散 （出自《永类钤方》）

组成： 白蔹、白术、白牵牛、白附子、白芷、白芍、白僵蚕各等分。

用法：除白僵蚕外，余药去皮或壳。7 药共研为粉末，贮瓶备用。每日早晚洗面。

功用：白面细肤。

七宝美髯丹（出自《本草纲目》引《积善堂方》）

组成：何首乌、茯苓、牛膝、当归、枸杞子、菟丝子、补骨脂。

用法：蜜丸，盐汤或酒下。

功用：治肝肾不足，须发早白。

健脑益智类名方举隅

七圣丸（出自《圣济总录》）

组成：茯苓、人参、天冬、远志、菖蒲、地骨皮、肉桂。

功用：益心志，令人聪明。

主治：心虚健忘。

养命开心益智方（出自《备急千金要方》）

组成：干地黄、人参、茯苓、肉苁蓉、远志、菟丝子、蛇床子。

功用：补肾，养心，益智。

主治：心肾虚，精血少，健忘失眠。

使用养身益寿方剂需要注意什么？

养身益寿药物虽有诸多益处，但进补时应当把握补益的原则与禁忌。清代名医程国彭云："补之为义，大矣哉！然有当补不补误人者；有不当补而补误人者；亦有当补而不分气血、不辨寒热、不分开合、不知缓急、不分五脏、不明根本，不深求调摄之方以误人者，是不可不讲也。"（《医学心悟》）具体应用时要根据不同年龄、性别、工作、生活环境、季节、体质特点进行补益。中医学认为虚证进补应遵循以下六个原则：辨证施补（辨体质用药、三因制宜）、不盲目进补、补勿过偏、盛者宜泻、泻不伤正、用药缓图。

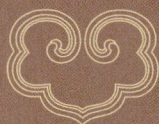

第七章

针灸养生

第一节
针灸养生概述

何谓针灸养生？

针灸养生就是采用针灸方法保健强身、防治疾病。"针"，即针刺。针刺疗法是根据脏腑经络学说，运用四诊八纲理论，结合辨病辨证体系，进行相应的配穴处方，按方施术，疏通经脉，调理气血，使阴阳归于相对平衡，达到防病治病效果的一种中医特色治疗方法。常用的针刺疗法有毫针刺法、火针疗法、电针疗法等。"灸"，是运用艾绒或其他药物在体表的穴位上燃烧，借灸火的热力以及药物的作用，通过经络的传导，以起到温经通络、温补元气、调和气血、祛寒暖宫的作用，从而达到防治疾病目的的一种中医特色治疗方法。

针灸养生的特点是什么？

一是历史悠久，实践经验丰富。二是疗效确切，操作简便易行，人们易于接受。三是常与其他保健方法配合使用，以增强效果。如针灸与气功、按摩结合，针灸与食疗结合，针灸与药物结合等。

第二节
针灸养生的机理

针灸养生的理论基础是什么？

针灸养生是以经络理论为基础的。人体经络系统由经脉和络脉组成，包括十二经脉、奇经八脉、十五络脉等。经络遍布全身，具有联系脏腑和肢体的作用，使人体脏腑、组织器官相互联系、有机配合，并有运行气血、濡养周身的作用。针灸是在一定的腧穴或经络路线上施术的，通过穴位、经络激发经络之气的功能，使人体新陈代谢旺盛起来，从而达到强壮身体、益寿延年的目的。

针灸的作用是什么？

一是扶正祛邪，增强机体免疫功能。针灸具有双向调节作用，既可补虚以扶正，又可泻实以祛邪。针刺保健与针刺治病的方法虽基本相同，但着眼点不同，针刺治病着眼于纠正机体阴阳、气血的偏盛偏衰，而针刺保健则着眼于强壮身体，增加机体代谢能力，旨在养生延寿。也正因为二者的着眼点不同，反映在选穴、用针上亦有一定差异。若用于保健，针刺手法刺激强度宜适中，选穴不宜多，且要以具有强壮功效的穴位为主。保健灸法是中国独特的养生方法之一，不仅可用于强身保健，也可用于久病体虚之人的康复。所谓保健灸法，就是在身体某些特定穴位上施灸，以达到和气血、调经络、养脏腑、延年益寿的目的。《医学入门》里说："药之不及，针之不到，必须灸之。"说明灸法可以起到针、药有时不能起到的作用。灸法的保健作用，早在《扁鹊心书》中就有明确的记载："人于无病时，常灸关元、气海、命门、中脘……虽未得长生，亦可保百余年寿矣。"

二是平衡阴阳，调整脏腑功能。阴阳平衡是健康者的生理状态，针灸养生的目的就是调整和维系这种状态。《灵枢·根结》云："用针之要，在于知调阴与阳，调阴与阳，精气乃光，合形与气，使神内藏。"说明针灸治疗疾病具有平衡阴阳、调整脏腑的作用。这种作用是通过经络阴阳属性、经穴配合和针灸手法来完成的。

三是疏通经络，调和气血。气血是人体生命活动的物质基础，依赖经络的传输布满全身，发挥推动、温煦、气化、巩固、防御、营养等作用。只有经络畅通，气血调和，脏腑功能才能正常进行，才能形泰而神安。通过一定的针灸手法，在腧穴部位进行适量的刺激，可以使阻塞的经络通畅而发挥其正常的生理功能，达到延年益寿的目的。

第三节
针灸养生应用

针刺疗法的适应证是什么？

针刺疗法可应用于以下疾病：神经系统疾病如特发性面神经麻痹、脑血管意外后遗症、运动神经元病、脊髓损伤等；各种神经痛如带状疱疹后神经痛、糖尿病周围神经病变所致的麻木疼痛、三叉神经痛等；运动系统疾病如颈椎病、腰椎病、骨关节病、肩周炎、急性扭伤等；内科疾病如类风湿性关节炎、强直性脊柱炎、慢性胃肠炎、肠易激综合征等；妇科疾病如月经病、卵巢早衰等；泌尿系统疾病如尿潴留、尿失禁等；五官科疾病如过敏性鼻炎、视神经萎缩等。此外，还适用于轻度焦虑抑郁、睡眠障碍、亚健康状态，以及减肥、美容等综合调理。

针刺疗法的禁忌证和注意事项是什么？

禁忌证：醉酒、情绪不稳或精神病患者；有传染性皮肤病或皮肤损伤者。

注意事项：接受治疗时不宜空腹或过饱；治疗后应注意保暖，避风寒，忌生冷。

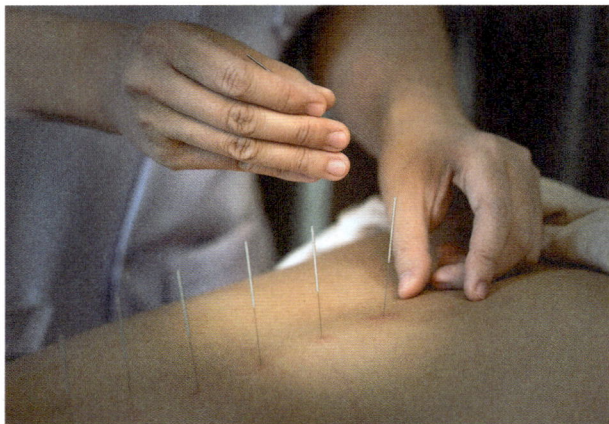

针刺操作

灸疗的适应证是什么？

灸疗可应用于以下疾病：寒凝血滞、经络痹阻所致的关节活动受限、肌肉僵硬；妇女寒凝经脉所致的痛经、月经不调；中焦虚寒所致的腹痛、泄泻、腹胀、便秘；肾阳虚所致阳痿遗精、失眠多梦、夜尿频数；疮疡久溃不愈；视神经萎缩；带状疱疹后神经痛。

灸疗的禁忌证和注意事项是什么？

禁忌证： 妊娠期妇女腰骶部、腹部不宜施灸。极度疲劳、过饥过饱、情绪不稳及醉酒者；艾叶过敏及易皮肤过敏者；属实热证或阴虚发热者不宜施灸。

注意事项： 艾灸后应避风寒；饭后不宜马上艾灸，以饭后1小时为宜；艾灸后不宜立即饮用凉水或进食生冷；艾灸后可能出现短暂疲劳感，此为正常现象，稍作休息即可缓解。

针灸常用保健穴位有哪些？

针灸常用保健穴位有合谷、足三里、风门、膏肓、关元、气海、神阙、大椎、涌泉等。

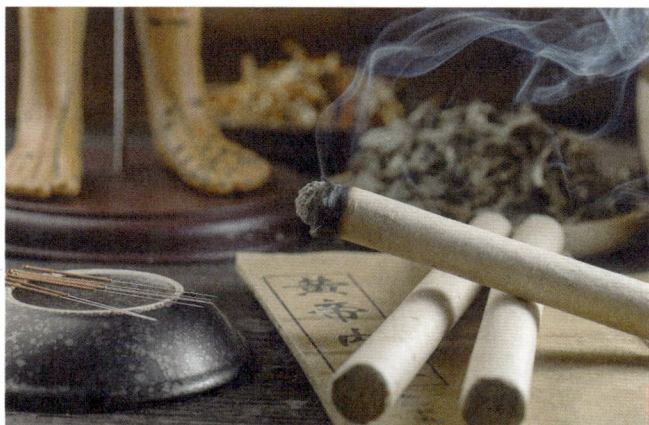

艾灸

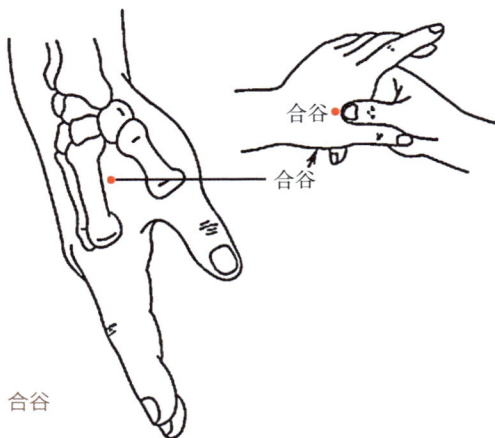

合谷

合谷

定位： 在手背，第1掌骨和第2掌骨之间，约平第2掌骨桡侧的中点。

功效： 醒脑开窍，疏风清热，镇痛通络。

操作： 直刺0.5～1寸。可灸。

防治病症： 头面五官疾病，热疒，无汗，自汗，盗汗，经闭，滞产，昏迷，癫病。

防治配伍： 补合谷，泻复溜可发汗；泻合谷，补复溜可止汗；配风池、大椎、曲池治外感发热；配下关、颊车治牙痛；配曲池、风市、膈俞治全身风疹。

足三里

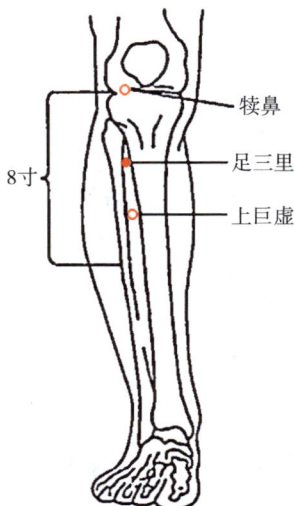

足三里

定位： 在小腿外侧，犊鼻下3寸，犊鼻与解溪连线上。

功效： 健脾和胃，调补气血，扶正培元。

操作： 直刺1～2寸。可灸。

防治病症： 胃痛，胃胀，呕吐，泄泻，便秘，高血压，神经衰弱，下肢痿痹。

防治配伍： 配内关、中脘治胃痛；配曲池、太冲治高血压；配曲池治荨麻疹；配水沟、内关、百会治休克。

常灸足三里不但能调理消化系统，防治胃肠疾病，且有强身保健，延年益寿之功效。

风门

定位：在背部，第 2 胸椎棘突下，后正中线旁开 1.5 寸。

功效：祛风解表，清热宣肺。

操作：直刺 0.5～1 寸。可灸。

防治病症：伤风咳嗽，头痛发热，荨麻疹，项强，腰背痛。

防治配伍：配大椎、肺俞、孔最治外感发热咳嗽；配风池、血海治荨麻疹；配风池、列缺治伤风头痛。

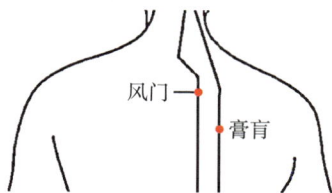

风门与膏肓

膏肓

定位：在背部，第 4 胸椎棘突下，后正中线旁开 3 寸。

功效：理肺气，补虚损。

操作：斜刺 0.5～0.8 寸。可灸。

防治病症：肺痨，咳喘，吐血，盗汗，脾胃虚弱，肩胛骨痛。

防治配伍：配关元、足三里加灸防治久病体弱羸瘦。

关元

定位：在下腹部，脐中下 4 寸，前正中线上。

功效：温肾固精，补气回阳，清热利湿。

操作：直刺 1～2 寸。孕妇禁针。

防治病症：腹痛，月经不调，带下，

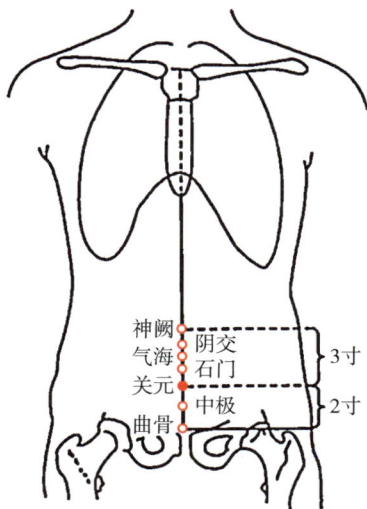

关元、气海与神阙

不孕，遗精，疝气，小便频数。

防治配伍： 配带脉、三阴交治白带过多；配三阴交、阴陵泉治遗精。

气海

定位： 在下腹部，脐中下1.5寸，前正中线上。

功效： 升补阳气，补虚固本。

操作： 直刺1～2寸。

防治病症： 小腹痛，月经不调，遗精，中风脱证，带下，崩漏，不孕，疝气，脱肛。

防治配伍： 配中极、肾俞、三阴交、行间治赤白带下；配归来治遗尿。

神阙

定位： 在上腹部，脐中央。

功效： 回阳救逆，健运脾胃。

操作： 禁针。艾条灸5～15min。

防治病症： 中风脱证，肠鸣，脱肛，泄泻不止，痢疾，腹痛。

防治配伍： 配足三里，治肠鸣腹痛；配长强、气海，治脱肛；配气海、阴陵泉，治疗泄利不止；配重灸关元，治疗中风脱证；神阙拔罐配刺天枢、足三里，治泄泻、呕吐。

大椎

定位： 在颈后部，第7颈椎棘突下凹陷中，后正中线上。

功效： 解表清热，清脑宁神。

操作： 向上斜刺0.5～1寸。

防治病症： 头项强痛，胸胁胀痛，肩背痛，头痛，发热，疟疾，癫痫，咳嗽，气喘。

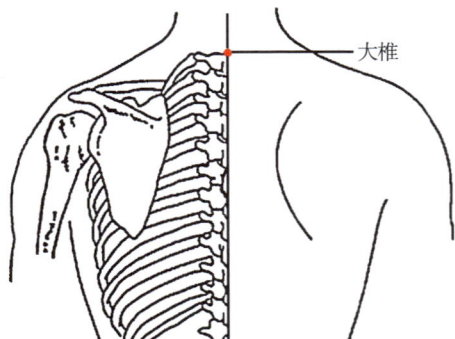

大椎

大椎

防治配伍：配曲池、合谷治流感；配丰隆治咳嗽；配足三里、曲池治白细胞减少。

涌泉

定位：在足底，屈足卷趾时足心最凹陷处。

功效：清热，开窍，宁神。

操作：直刺 0.5 ~ 1 寸。

防治病症：头痛，头昏，中风昏迷，休克，小儿惊风，小便不利，大便难，足心热痛。

防治配伍：配关元、丰隆治虚劳咳嗽；配水沟治小儿惊风；配足三里治中毒性休克；配昆仑治大便难。

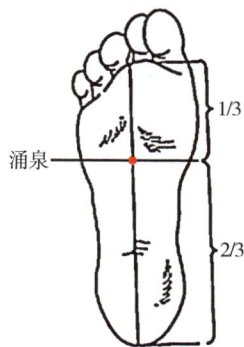

涌泉

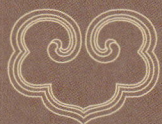

第八章

其他非药物

养生方法

第一节
非药物疗法概述

中医非药物疗法的优势是什么？

中医非药物疗法是中国传统医学的重要组成部分，是劳动人民长期和疾病作斗争的经验总结，其内容丰富、范围广泛、历史悠久，经过历代医家的不懈努力和探索，取得了巨大成就。中医非药物疗法在未病先防、既病防变方面具有很大优势，体现了传统医学治未病、防重于治、养生保健和健康调养的学术思想。中医非药物疗法历经数千年坎坷不平的发展，充分显现了自己顽强的生命力和强大的优势所在：一是疗效可靠、迅速、显著；二是传统医学疗法适应证广泛，可用于临床各科数百种疾病的治疗和预防保健；三是安全性较好，由于皮肤、黏膜屏障的自我保护功能及使用的多为天然药物，使得外治法极少有毒副作用；四是减少了内服药物之苦。

什么是非药物养生疗法？

非药物养生疗法不借助内服药物，通过行之有效的养生保健方法，起到健身美容、宁神益智、防病祛疾、延年益寿的作用。

非药物养生疗法种类多样，常见的有针灸、推拿、按摩、气功、导引、拔罐、砭疗、火疗、中药熏蒸、药浴、蜡疗、贴敷等。

非药物养生疗法的应用禁忌是什么？

有下列情况之一者，不宜进行非药物养生疗法：情绪急躁，七情（喜、怒、忧、思、悲、恐、惊）过激时；病情起伏较大，高热、神志不清，有并发症趋势，病情恶化，病重病危阶段；过饥、过饱、酒醉后；妊娠期、月经期；雷电交加、狂风暴雨、烈日曝晒时；空气污染、居地潮湿，嘈杂不安的环境；身体疲乏或极度虚弱时；精神失常、不能控制行为时；房事前后。

非药物养生疗法的选择原则是什么？

在众多的方法中，应根据个人体质的类型，身体的强弱，并参考职业、年龄、性别、爱好等来选择。至于因防治疾病而进行的非药物疗法，则除了考虑以上种种因素外，还要辨别证候的属性和疾病的特点，因人施术、辨证施术、辨病施术。

第二节
按摩导引

按摩的基本手法有哪些?

按摩的基本手法有拍打法、叩击法、抚摩法、旋摩法、点按法、指揉法、掌揉法、指捏法、掌搓法、剁掌法、推导法、抓拿法、抖动法。

按摩导引术式有哪些?

按摩导引的术式多样,常见的有老子按摩法、天竺国按摩法、气功按摩十八法、淹城引导术、马王堆导引术、五禽戏、八段锦、太极拳、虾蟆行气法、广渡导引术、龟鳖行气法、雁行气法、龙行气法等。

第三节
养生气功

什么是气功？

气功是中医养生学的一个重要组成部分。它是练功者通过调身、调心、调息来发挥自身内在潜能，达到增强体质、祛病延年的一种保健方法。

气功的练习要领是什么？

气功的练习要领是松静自然、意气合一、动静相兼、上虚下实、辨证练功、练养相兼、循序渐进。

气功练习的基本方法是什么？

气功的流派很多，但不外静功、动功、动静结合功三大类。锻炼的基本方法概括起来有调身（姿势）、调心（意念）、调息（呼吸）三大法。

如何调身？

调身是指调整身体姿势、松弛躯体，以正确的动作锻炼身体。不论何种功法，都讲究姿势，正确的姿势既有劲而又能放得松，所谓"筋骨要弓，肌肉要松，节节贯串，虚灵其中"，这样可使周身气血运行通畅，为顺利进行调心、调息创造条件。

如何调心？

调心是指意念训练，即在练功中要求自己的思想情绪、意识意念等通过训练而逐步进入空虚入静状态，进而达到能以意领气，意气合一，调动机体潜能。

如何调息？

调息是指呼吸的调整和锻炼。调整呼吸不仅可以直接调和气血，锻炼内脏，也可以积蓄和运行内气。调息要做到匀、缓、细、长、自然，概括起来有自然呼吸法、腹式呼吸法、停闭式呼吸法、大呼吸法、风呼吸法、踵息法、胎息法、休息法和读字呼吸法。

常用气功功法有哪些?

气功常用功法包括放松功、站桩功、内养功、周天功、睡功、意气功、虚名功、易筋洗髓经、混元易筋经、六字诀等。

第四节
中医养生适宜技术

何谓砭疗？

砭疗是用石质工具对体表皮肤的特定部位反复进行刮拭，从而起到解表祛邪、清热解毒、活血化瘀、舒筋活络作用的一种中医特色治疗方法。

砭疗的器具有哪些？

《说文解字》："砭，以石刺病也。"用于治病的石头称为砭石或砭具，是人类最早使用的医疗器械。目前常用的砭具依照对人体的作用、功能分为按摩砭具、温熨砭具和割刺、罐疗砭具。

砭疗的适应证是什么？

砭疗的适应证有：软组织损伤类疾病，如急性或慢性腰扭伤、肌肉拉伤、膝关节脂肪垫劳损等；骨伤类疾病，如颈椎病、腰椎间盘突出或腰椎管狭窄引起的坐骨神经痛、退行性骨关节炎、网球肘等；风湿类疾病，如风湿及类风湿性关节炎、肩周炎、膝关节滑膜炎等；周围神经病，如周围性面瘫、面肌痉挛、末梢神经炎、慢性神经疾病导致的肌肉萎缩等；心血管疾病，如心肌缺血、心律不齐等；各种功能性失调，如慢性疲劳、失眠、神经衰弱等。还可用于美容及减肥。

砭疗的禁忌证和注意事项是什么？

禁忌证：出血倾向疾病，如血小板减少症、白血病、严重贫血等；危重病症，如急性传染病、重症心脏病等；皮肤有损伤、炎症、溃烂或疮疡初愈。饱食或饥饿，以及对砭疗恐惧者不宜进行砭疗。

注意事项：头部不使用叩法；心脏附近不使用叩法和振法；孕妇腹部不做砭术治疗；老弱者慎用凉法；对老弱者和人体脆弱部位要慎重掌握施术的力度；使用温法时勿因温度过高而造成皮肤的烫伤。

何谓火疗？

火疗是将不同作用的中药贴敷于体表穴位和患部，利用酒精燃烧的热力和空气对流的原理，通过经络刺激和中药透皮吸收，起到调和阴阳、温经通脉、行气活血作用的一种中医特色治疗方法。

火疗的适应证是什么？

火疗的适应证有：风寒湿痹所致的急性或慢性疼痛；颈、腰椎疾病所致的局部疼痛、麻木；骨关节病所致的关节疼痛；肌肉劳损、软组织损伤所致的各种疼痛；妇女寒凝经脉所致的痛经、月经不调；阳虚所致的失眠多梦、四肢不温、夜尿频多；脾肾虚寒所致的腹痛、便溏、便秘。

火疗的禁忌证和注意事项是什么？

禁忌证：严重疾病患者如恶性肿瘤、高血压控制不佳、肾功能衰竭、出血倾向等。醉酒、情绪不稳者，精神病患者，有传染性皮肤病或皮肤损伤者，以及妊娠妇女不宜进行火疗。

注意事项：不宜空腹火疗，饭后1小时为宜；进行火疗前应摘除身上的金属饰品以防烫伤；火疗后应注意保暖，避风寒、忌生冷。

什么是中药熏蒸疗法？

中药熏蒸疗法是用不同作用的中草药煎煮产生的药气熏蒸人体不同部位，通过皮肤、孔窍直达病所，经过玄府开阖将体内的湿浊排出体外，起到祛湿排毒、调理阴阳、温经通络作用的一种中医特色治疗方法。

中药熏蒸疗法的适应证是什么？

中药熏蒸疗法的适应证有：脂质代谢异常；纤维肌痛综合征；关节肿胀、疼痛及活动受限；腰肌劳损、软组织挫伤、筋膜炎、肌腱炎；睡眠障碍、轻度焦虑抑郁；肥胖及亚健康状态。

中药熏蒸疗法的禁忌证和注意事项是什么？

禁忌证：严重疾病如恶性肿瘤、血压控制不佳、肾功能衰竭、出血倾向等。有传染性皮肤病或皮肤损伤者，妊娠期及月经期妇女不宜进行中药气疗。

注意事项：年老体弱者熏蒸时间不宜过长，需家属陪同；注意保暖、避风寒、忌生冷。

何谓药浴？

药浴是通过中医辨证，根据不同的疾病，加入不同药物，利用水温对皮肤、经络、穴位的刺激和药物的透皮吸收，达到治疗疾病、养生保健作用的一种中医特色治疗方法。

药浴的适应证是什么？

药浴的适应证有：风寒湿痹所致的关节及肌肉疼痛、肌炎、皮肌炎等；各种原因所致的失眠；高脂血症；糖尿病足；干燥综合征；硬皮病、牛皮癣、湿疹。

药浴的禁忌证和注意事项是什么？

禁忌证：高血压、低血压、心脏功能不全；皮肤有较大面积创口。经期女性及孕妇，以及具有严重过敏史的患者不宜进行药浴。

注意事项：不宜空腹药浴，饭后1小时为宜；药浴期间应适当补充水分；药浴后应避风寒，忌生冷；每次浸泡时间不宜太长，身体虚弱者在浸泡过程中可能会出现头晕、心率加快、恶心、全身酸软无力等症状，应停止药浴，稍作休息。

何谓蜡疗？

蜡疗是将具有不同作用的中药药粉与加热的医用石蜡混合敷在患部，借助石蜡柔和温热的特性，辅助中药进行局部刺激与透皮吸收，二者结合，起到温经通脉、行气活血作用的一种中医特色治疗方法。

蜡疗的适应证是什么？

蜡疗的适应证有：颈、腰椎疾病所致的局部麻木、疼痛；骨关节病所致的关节僵硬疼痛；肌肉劳损、软组织损伤所致的僵硬、疼痛；风寒湿痹所致的慢性疼痛；妇女寒凝经脉所致的痛经、月经不调。

蜡疗的禁忌证和注意事项是什么？

禁忌证：严重疾病如恶性肿瘤、高血压控制不佳、肾功能衰竭、出血倾向等；醉酒、情绪不稳者或精神病患者，有传染性皮肤病或皮肤损伤者不宜进行蜡疗。

注意事项：不宜空腹及过饱状态下治疗；蜡疗后应注意保暖，避风寒、忌生冷。

何谓推拿？

推拿是指医生运用自己的双手作用于患者体表、受伤部位、不适所在、特定腧穴，运用推、拿、按、摩、揉、捏、点、拍等形式多样的手法，以达到疏通经络、推行气血、扶伤止痛、祛邪扶正、调和阴阳作用的一种中医特色治疗方法。

推拿的适应证是什么？

推拿的适应证有：软组织损伤、关节扭伤所致关节肌肉疼痛；骨质增生、颈椎病、椎间盘突出、肩周炎等；头痛、头晕、高血压、胃炎、糖尿病等；月经不调、痛经、闭经、乳腺炎等；脾胃虚寒所致腹泻、便秘。

推拿的禁忌证和注意事项是什么？

禁忌证：急性或慢性传染病、皮肤病、出血性疾病；恶性肿瘤、严重的高血压、心脏病；骨折初期、脱臼及严重外伤；严重的骨质疏松、颈腰部椎体滑脱。

注意事项：推拿后应避风寒，忌生冷，适量饮用温水补充机体水分；过饥过饱均不宜推拿，饭后1小时为宜。

TCM Health
Preservation

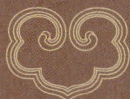

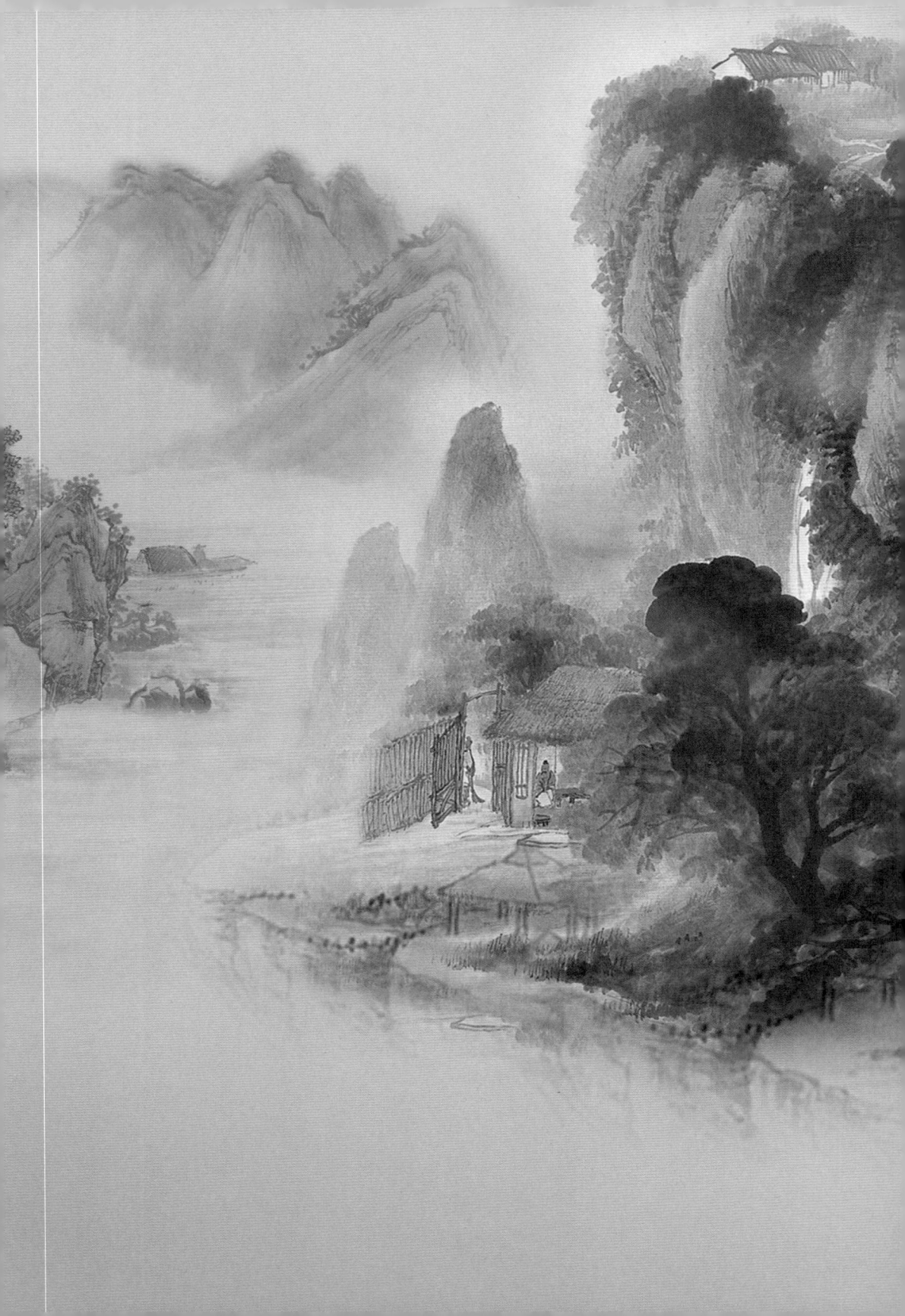

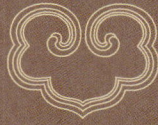

Chapter 1

A Brief History of TCM

Health Preservation

When did TCM health preservation originate?

The origin of TCM health preservation can be traced back to before the Spring and Autumn Period. Although in a primitive society where productivity was extremely low and ancient human beings lived a life of eating and drinking blood, as an instinctive need, human beings were promoted to explore ways to alleviate illnesses and prolong life. In the unearthed oracle bone inscriptions of the Yin-Shang Dynasty, there are words presenting the pursuit of hygiene, such as "Mù (shower)" and "Yù (bath)", which shows that as early as the 14th century BC, China had already taken measures to preserve health and prevent diseases. By the end of primitive society, people had already known how to use exercises and sports to treat and prevent diseases. For example, *Master Lv's Spring and Autumn Annals–Ancient Music* recorded: "In ancient times, at the beginning of Taotang's governance, there was a lot of stagnant yin energy that accumulated, causing blockage in the waterways and hindering its natural flow. The people's spirits were depressed and stagnant, and their curled-up tendons and bones could not stretch, so the dance was created to guide the flow of qi." The so-called "dance" is the embryonic form of daoyin therapy to activate the joints and make the circulation of qi and blood smooth. *Biography of Immortals* and other literatures also recorded that Peng Zu in ancient times lived 800 years because of his way of health preservation. From today's point of view, it is impossible for people to live 800 years old, but at least it shows that people paid attention to the way of health preservation as early as ancient times. A dialogue between Qi Bo and Huangdi mentioned that "the ancient people who knew Tao...passed away after 100 years old" (*Basic Questions–Shanggu Tianzhen Lun*), in which "Tao" refers to the health preservation method today. However, before the Spring and Autumn Period, a complete medical system had not yet been formed, and the treatment methods were very primitive, so health preservation before the Spring and Autumn Period was still in its infancy. The characteristics of health preservation in this period are conforming to nature, and focusing on dietetic aftercare and exercises.

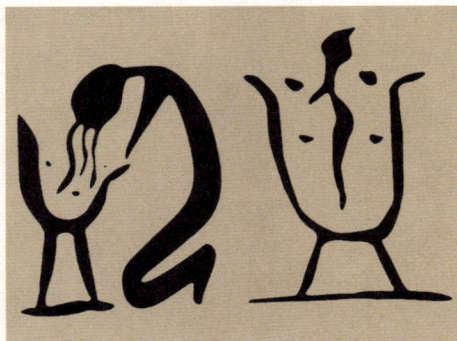

"Mù (shower)" (left) and "Yù (bath)" (right) in inscriptions on bones or tortoise shells of the Shang Dynasty

How did Taoist thoughts dominate the formation of TCM health preservation?

Taoism generally refers to the philosophical schools centering on the theories of Laozi and Zhuangzi in the pre-Qin period. It is generally believed that Laozi is the founder of Taoism. Laozi, also known as Li Er, lived in the Spring and Autumn Period. His masterpiece is *Tao Te Ching*, and his academic thought basically belongs to naturalistic philosophy. Zhuang Zhou in the Warring States Period, inherited and carried forward Laozi's thoughts. Taoism in this period is also called "Lao-Zhuang philosophy". The word "yangsheng (health preservation)" first appeared in *Zhuangzi*, in which health preservation was especially discussed in *The Key to Health Preservation*. *Zhuangzi–Keyi* said "Breathing to exhale the turbid qi and inhale fresh air, climbing the tree like a bear, and sprawling like a bird are all for the best of longevity", which is the exposition of his health-preserving thought. The "Tao" advocated by Taoism refers to the essence of all things in heaven and earth and the natural laws of their cycles. Everything in the natural world is in constant motion and change, and Tao is the fundamental principle governing it. The *Tao Te Ching* states: "Man follows the earth, earth follows heaven, heaven follows the Tao, and the Tao follows nature." This is a specific exposition on the concept of Tao. Therefore, human activities should conform to the laws of nature in order to achieve longevity. This is the fundamental idea of Taoist thought. The ideas of tranquility, inaction, returning to simplicity, conforming to nature, valuing softness, and achieving harmony have had a great influence on the field of TCM and health preservation. The influence of Taoism on TCM health preservation is mainly reflected in the following aspects: first, the basic concepts such as essence, qi and spirit were put forward; second, the static regimen was established; third, it worships nature, so the qigong health preservation method that conforms to nature was created; fourth, valuing softness is advocated; fifth, the significance and principles of health preservation were expounded philosophically.

In exploring the history of health preservation and learning health-preserving techniques, the influence of Taoism cannot be ignored. However, it is important to note that early Taoist methods of health preservation, such as those of Laozi and Zhuangzi, contain passive ideas of conforming to nature, and these should be rectified in specific research and practice.

How did Confucianism promote the formation of TCM health preservation theory?

Confucianism, represented by Confucius and Mencius, has always been the backbone of ancient Chinese intellectual history. It is also the "way of governance" ruled by the feudal society for thousands of years, which has had a profound influence on China's politics and culture, as well as medicine. In the history of medicine, there is a saying that "there is no distinction between medicine and Confucianism". Confucianism takes the "doctrine of the mean" as the method of self-cultivation, and Confucius, the originator of Confucianism, was the advocate and practitioner of health preservation. Therefore, the Confucian health preservation method enriched TCM health preservation and promoted the formation of its theory.

The "mean and harmony view" in Confucianism has the deepest influence on TCM health preservation, which is discussed explicitly in *The Doctrine of the Mean*. *The Records of the Grand Historian–The Hereditary House of Confucius* states: "Zisi authored *The Doctrine of the Mean*". Zisi, also known as Kong Ji, was Confucius' grandson. Confucius' thought on mean and harmony was preserved and recorded by him. The so-called "doctrine of the mean" is a state of human nature cultivation in Confucianism—"harmony without going adrift" and "mean without partial opinions", which is neither too much nor too little. *The Doctrine of the Mean* said that "mean refers to not showing anger, sorrows or joys; harmony refers to controlling the emotions in an appropriate way if they are shown. Mean and harmony are the fundamental nature of the world. Harmony is the principle that everyone should follow. Once the mean and harmony are reached, the world will return to its position, and everything will prosper". That is to say, as long as people's self-cultivation reaches the state of the mean and harmony, the effect of "the world will return to its position, and everything will prosper" will be produced. When discussing the reasons for the longevity of ancient people, *The Yellow Emperor's Inner Classic* (most commonly known as *Huangdi Neijing*) pointed out that "the ancient people who knew the law of health preservation could abide by the law of yin and yang to harmonize the way of health preservation". The word "harmonize" is probably the earliest record of the Confucian concept of the mean and harmony view applied to health preservation, that is, to achieve the state of harmony through health preservation.

In this way, yin is not deficient and yang is not hyperactive, and people "died after a hundred years old". Later doctors also mentioned the health preservation theory of "harmony" time after time in their works, which shows its deep influence.

Confucian thought enriched the content of TCM health preservation and promoted the formation of TCM health preservation theories. Its main academic ideas and concepts include three key points:

The first point is the emphasis on mental regulation. Confucius attached great importance to spiritual health preservation, advocated self-cultivation, and paid attention to moral cultivation. Mencius paid more attention to "heart nourishment". "If getting enough nourishment, everything will grow; if losing nourishment, everything will fade" (*Mencius–Gaozi Part One*); the specific method of heart nourishment is "For mind cultivation, there is nothing better than having few desire. Although there are people who lose their heart among those with few desire, the number is small" (*Mencius–Jinxin Part Two*). As a result, later Confucian representatives Dong Zhongshu, Cheng Yi, Zhu Xi and doctor Sun Simiao made further development, and connected it with health preservation methods, forming a health preservation school with Confucian characteristics. Confucius also put forward the idea of "three precepts", saying that "a gentleman has three precepts: when he is young and his blood and qi are unstable, he should be cautious of sexual seduction; when he reaches the prime of his life and his blood and qi are strong, he should be cautious of fight; when he is old and his blood and qi are declining, he should be cautious of greediness" (*The Analects of Confucius–Jishi*).

The second point is the emphasis on physical care. This is a concrete manifestation of the Confucian concept of "mean and harmony". Regular daily routines, balanced work and rest, and moderate diet are basic principles for maintaining the body. Under the influence of the Confucian health preservation thought of "mean and harmony", rich theory, principles, and methods of health preservation were formed. For example, in the Song Dynasty, Yan Yonghe's *Formulas to Aid the Living* states: "Those skilled in health preservation are cautious about balance and moderation. Every drink and meal should enter the stomach and be digested and transformed promptly, avoiding the risk of stagnation. If one is inherently weak and eats irregularly, or excessively consuming fishy foods, dairy, cold fruits and vegetables, it will cause accumulation in the stomach, leading to chronic stagnation." This reflects the influence of Confucian dietary balance. Additionally, there are words like "Those who achieve harmony and balance will surely live long", in *YangXing Yanming Lu* and "Human life is like the heaven and earth; when harmonious, it is spring, when gloomy, it is autumn" in *Yishu*.

Third, Confucius had unique views on dietetic health preservation. For example, regarding dietetic hygiene, Confucius put forward that "never get tired of finely-ground grain, and never get tired of finely-cut meat. If the grains, meat and fish are rotten and stinky, one should not eat them. Do not eat it if the color of the food is bad; do not eat it if the food is not cooked well; do not eat it if it is not the proper time to eat" (*The Analects of Confucius–Xiangdang*). Many of the later generations' views on dietetic health preservation have developed from Confucius' original ideas on dietetic health preservation, such as "eating fine food can nourish people, while eating coarse food can harm people" (*The Essays of Tui'an*), "It is appropriate to eat when you are hungry, and you can never get tired of carefully chewing. Don't wait till you are extremely thirsty before you drink, and you can never get tired of carefully sipping" (*Appropriate Diet*).

The Confucian health preservation philosophy, particularly the Confucian view of "mean and harmony", has been followed by physicians throughout history and has significantly influenced the development of health preservation practices in later generations. Even today, it still holds practical value.

How does *Huangdi Neijing* influence TCM health preservation?

Before *Huangdi Neijing*, health preservation was in the experimental stage, and there was no systematic health preservation theory. It comprehensively absorbed the achievements of health preservation studies prior to the Qin and Han Dynasties, and provided a relatively thorough and systematic discussion of the theories, methods, and principles related to TCM's health preservation. Therefore, in the history of TCM health preservation, the completion of the *Huangdi Neijing* is a milestone, which laid a theoretical foundation for the formation of TCM health preservation.

The contribution of *Huangdi Neijing* to TCM health preservation is mainly reflected in the following aspects:

First, it emphasized the three treasures of the human body: essence, qi and spirit. According to the *Huangdi Neijing*, the essence is the basic substance that constitutes the human body. "When people are born, the essence is formed first, and then the brain marrow is formed" (*Miraculous Pivot–Meridians*). At the same time, the essence is the original motive force of human life activities, and it is the origin of strength and longevity. "The essence is the foundation of the body" (*Basic Questions–Jingui Zhenyan Lun*). Qi refers to subtle essential substances and the ability of viscera activities. The end of a person's life is when "all the five internal organs are empty, and all the qi and spirit are gone, leaving the body alone and dead" (*Miraculous Pivot–Tiannian*). Spirit is the general name of life activity phenomenon, and it is the concentrated expression of all life activities such as spirit, consciousness, perception and movement. "Those who have spirit will prosper, while those who lose spirit die" (*Basic Questions–Yijing Bianqi Lun*). It can be seen that essence, qi and spirit are the three most precious treasures of the human body, so experts in health preservation of later generations paid more attention to nourishing essence, invigorating qi and adjusting spirit.

Second, the principle of "correspondence between human body and natural environment" was established. *Huangdi Neijing* views human and the natural world as an integrated whole, meaning that as changes occur in nature, corresponding responses occur in human. *Huangdi Neijing* holds that the gist of health preservation is "adapting to the four seasons and different weathers, living in peace with emotions and being satisfied with the residences, controlling yin and yang and adjusting rigidity and softness" (*Miraculous Pivot–Benshen*), and puts forward the famous principle of health preservation in four seasons "nourishing yang in spring and summer, and nourishing yin in autumn and winter". *Basic Questions–Shanggu Tianzhen Lun* explicitly states "avoiding the deceptive and harmful winds in a timely manner", thereby pioneering the prevention and treatment of diseases.

Third, it explains the laws of life. *Huangdi Neijing* provides insightful observations and scientific summaries of the life cycle stages of birth, growth, maturity, aging, and death in the human body. *Miraculous Pivot–Tiannian* divided people's growth and development into ten stages, each of which was ten years. *Basic Questions–Yinyang Yingxiang Dalun* also basically adopted the ten-year division method. However, *Basic Questions–Shanggu Tianzhen Lun* took seven years for women and eight years for men as the cycle. These are the earliest in the history of Chinese medicine regarding the classification of human growth, development, and aging cycles. They provide a reference for future research in TCM on the laws of life and geriatrics in preventing aging and promoting longevity.

Fourth, it established the theory of meridians, which laid the theoretical foundation for non-pharmaceutical health therapies such as qigong, daoyin, and massage. The silk manuscripts unearthed in Mawangdui, Changsha, *Moxibustion Classic of Eleven Foot-Arm Meridians* and *Moxibustion Classic of Eleven Yin-Yang Meridians*, although written earlier than *Huangdi Neijing*, are simple in content and do not establish systematic meridian theory. *Huangdi Neijing* formed a systematic and complete meridian theory, which included twelve meridians, eight extra meridians, etc., and pointed out that the function of meridians is "to promote blood and qi and nourish yin and yang, nurture tendons and bones, and lubricate joints" (*Miraculous Pivot–Benzang*).

Fifth, it summarized and preserved many effective methods and principles of health preservation before the Warring States Period. For example, "being indifferent to fame or gain, the genuine qi will follow the direction, and the essence and spirit are kept inside" is the summary of Taoist spirit perservation methods. In addition, effective principles and methods for health preservation were proposed, such as health preserving with food and dietetic therapy, integration of motion and stillness, and physical exercises.

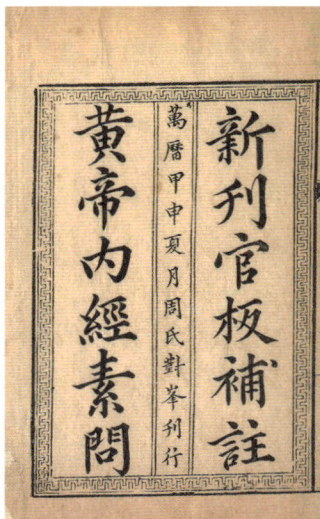

Huangdi Neijing made great contributions to TCM health preservation, which firmly laid the theoretical foundation of TCM health preservation. Although TCM health preservation has been improved in theory and innovated in methods, it is always under of guidance of *Huangdi Neijing*.

The Yellow Emperor's Inner Classic Basic Questions (Huáng Dì Nèi Jīng Sù Wèn, 黄帝内经素问)

How did exhalation-inhalation and daoyin therapy promote the development of health preservation?

Huangdi Neijing summarized the sprouting and spreading of exhalation-inhalation and daoyin therapy. It established that the important measure for ancient people to "live to an expected longevity and die after a hundred years old" is "to harmonize the ways of health preservation", and the exhalation-inhalation and daoyin therapy is among one of the ways. The mechanism of exhalation-inhalation and daoyin therapy to deter the disease is that "the genuine qi will follow the direction, and the essence and spirit are kept inside", and the main methods of daoyin therapy are to adjust the spirit (heart), adjust the qi (breath) and adjust the body, that is, "regulate breathing and absorb pure clear qi; be detached and alone, and keep the spirit inside; exercise the body, so that the tendons, bones and muscles are highly coordinated with the whole body" (*Basic Questions–Shanggu Tianzhen Lun*).

During the Warring States Period, due to the rise of Taoism, the exhalation-inhalation and daoyin therapy in this period, and even the qigong afterwards, had a distinct feature. That is, they were combined with the Taoist thought of "quietness and inaction".

The daoyin therapy in the Han Dynasty and the Three Kingdoms Period was inherited from that in the Warring States Period and the Qin Dynasty, but it was innovated in theory and method. Zhang Zhongjing also placed great importance on daoyin and tuna, advocating for using physical movement and breathing techniques to prevent and treat illnesses. For example, he stated: "As soon as the limbs feel heavy and sluggish, practice daoyin and tuna...Do not let the nine orifices become obstructed" (*Synopsis of Golden Chamber*). In the Eastern Han Dynasty, Wang Chong and Hua Tuo made some supplements and exertions to the theory of health preservation in the *Huangdi Neijing*, which promoted the development of exhalation-inhalation and daoyin therapy. In *Discussion of Balance*, Wang Chong specifically explored issues related to health and longevity in nearly twenty chapters, discussing topics such as life and death, longevity and premature death, and methods for extending life. For example, the *Discussion of Balance–Qishou* said: "If a person has abundant qi, he will have a strong body; if he is strong, he will have a long life. If a person lacks qi, he will be weak; if he is weak, he will have a short life." It clearly put forward the view that those with strong innate endowments would have longer life spans, while those with weak innate endowments would live shorter lives. And in *Zi Ji*, it is recorded: "Nurture your energy and maintain self-discipline, drink wine in moderation. Close your eyes and ears to distractions, cherish and preserve your essence. Appropriately supplement with medicine and practice daoyin, in hopes of extending life and staying youthful for a long time." This documents some of his own methods for "nurturing energy and self-discipline" and "using medicine and daoyin". Xun Yue, a historian at the end of the Han Dynasty, said in *Shen Jian–Suxian* that "two inches adjacent to the umbilicus is called the barrier, and Taoists often cause qi to pass, which is for the requirement". It is proof that the relationship between qigong and meridians and acupoints was already noticed at that time, and there had been such exercises as qi penetrating Guanyuan and keeping the idea in Guanyuan. Hua Tuo was a famous physician who lived at the same time as Zhang Zhongjing. He inherited the idea that "running water will not stink, and the door shaft that often rotates will not rot" put forward in *Master Lv's Spring and Autumn Annals*, and further explained the principle of exercise health preservation in theory. *Romance of The Three Kindoms–Biograpy of Huatuo* recorded: "The human body needs constant exercise, but it must not be excessive. When the human body moves, the nutrients in food can be digested, and the blood vessels are unobstructed, so people will not get sick, just like the door is always open and closed, so the door pivot does not rot." He also inherited the rule of "exhaling the old and inhaling the new like bears climbing and birds stretching" in *Zhuangzi*, and created Wuqinxi (The Five Animal Frolics) of exercise health preservation. Wuqinxi is an exercise that imitates the movements of five animals: tiger, deer, bear, monkey, and bird. The tiger frolic is vigorous and powerful, embodying strength and might; regular practice can make the limbs strong and enhance physical power. The deer frolic features fluid movements with a balance of motion and stillness; regular practice can make the waist and legs flexible, promote a natural demeanor, and improve physical appearance. The bear frolic involves steady and firm steps, embodying the strength to move mountains; regular practice can enhance resilience and endurance. The monkey frolic is characterized by agility and swift movements, with playful gestures like rubbing the face; regular practice can keep the mind clear, improve reflexes, and make movements light. The bird frolic mimics the carefree flight of birds in the sky, with movements that rise and fall gracefully; regular practice can make the body light and agile. Over time, Wuqinxi has evolved to not only prevent and treat diseases but also to improve overall physical fitness, advancing the practice of guiding and conducting exercises.

In the Wei, Jin and Northern and Southern Dynasties, the theory, content and methods of daoyin therapy were further developed. Ji Kang's *Health Preservation Theory* involved a lot of contents of daoyin, and expounded that "proper application of daoyin health preservation can help one live up to his life". There are many of Ge Hong's incisive expositions on qigong in *Bao Pu Zi*. He pointed out that the function of qigong was to "nourish the body inside and dispel the pathogen outside", and the mechanism of daoyin therapy was to "diffuse nutrient qi and defensive qi". He also advocated that daoyin therapy should be both dynamic and static, not limited to forms. "Either flexing or stretching, looking down or up, walking or lying, or leaning and standing, or lingering, or pacing, or chanting, or sighing, all belong to daoyin." It had a certain influence on the diversification of the forms of daoyin therapy in later generations. There was also a Taoist priest named Xu Xun in the Jin Dynasty. His book, *Records of Jingming Religion*, also recorded some daoyin methods. Especially the word "qigong" in "if qigong is successfully practised, the bones and tendons are harmonized and soft, and the hundreds of passes are unobstructed" may probably be the earliest record of the word "qigong" in the existing literature.

In the Sui and Tang Dynasties, daoyin therapy was officially recognized by the imperial court and determined as a means of health preservation and medical treatment. Due to the recognition of the imperial court and the accumulation of long-term practice, the development of daoyin therapy in the Sui and Tang Dynasties reached its peak. Among the 1,729 diseases discussed in the *General Treatise on Causes and Manifestations of All Diseases* by Chao Yuanfang, a doctor (an ancient medical teaching professional title) of imperial doctors in the Sui Dynasty, only the method of "practicing daoyin to nourish and supplement" was supported by concrete, vivid and effective explanations in almost every disease. Other therapies and methods were either briefly described or not described at all. Sun Simiao, a great doctor in the Tang Dynasty, is also an expert in health preservation who paid great attention to daoyin. He recorded a lot of contents related to daoyin and activating qi in *Essential Recipes for Emergent Use Worth A Thousand Gold* and *Prescriptions for Health*

Preservation Hidden in Pillows. In addition, some contents of Buddhist exercises were also recorded in *Essential Recipes for Emergent Use Worth A Thousand Gold*, indicating that many schools of exhalation-inhalation and daoyin therapy coexisted in this period.

In a word, after the continuous accumulation and development in the Spring and Autumn Period, the Warring States Period, the Qin and Han Dynasties, the Wei, Jin and Northern and Southern Dynasties, the exhalation-inhalation and daoyin therapy sprouted in the primitive times became an important part of TCM health preservation in the Sui and Tang Dynasties, and has been continuously popularized and improved.

What are the schools of TCM health preservation?

With the completion of *Huangdi Neijing*, TCM health preservation ushered in the first peak in its development history during the Warring States Period. The thoughts of Taoism and Confucianism also infiltrated into health preservation, grafted with health preservation theory, and initially formed different styles of health preservation viewpoints and methods.

For the convenience of research and inheritance, the TCM health preservation schools can be divided into Taoist health preservation school, Buddhist health preservation school, Confucian health preservation school, and doctor health preservation school by the method of dividing schools in medical history. There is no strict boundaries among all schools. Especially in the Tang Dynasty, Confucianism, Buddhism and Taoism had the trend of "three religions in one", and many health preservation experts and health preservation works were eclectic and permeated mutually.

What are the characteristics of Taoist health preservation school?

Since the Qin Dynasty, Taoism has first gotten attention. Many scholars and alchemists, such as Zhang Liang, Li Shaojun and Dongfang Shuo, who believed in Lao-Zhuang philosophy, strongly advocated health preservation methods such as daoyin and exhalation-inhalation. Ji Kang wrote *Health Preservation Theory*, which reiterated the health preservation theory and method of Taoism. Ge Hong wrote *Bao Pu Zi*, which extensively discussed various Taoist health preservation theories and methods, so that the orthodox Taoist health preservation techniques can be systematically developed. If Laozi and Zhuangzi can be called the founders of the Taoist health preservation school, Ge Hong is its representative figure without doubt.

What are the characteristics of Buddhist health preservation school?

Buddhism originated in India and was later introduced to Xinjiang of China through Central Asia. It was introduced to China's mainland in the late Western Han Dynasty (according to the *Outline of Chinese History* edited by Jian Bozan). After Buddhism was introduced into China, it was first juxtaposed with the theories of Huangdi and Laozi, and there was a folk saying that "when Laozi came to Dongyi, he became the Buddha". Therefore, although Buddhist health preservation methods spread with the introduction of Buddhism, they were mostly attached to Taoist health preservation methods in the early days and did not develop greatly. It was not until the Sui and Tang Dynasties that it began to rise suddenly and became independent as a school of health preservation. Sun Simiao's *Essential Recipes for Emergent Use Worth A Thousand Gold* included the massage and daoyin method of ancient Tianzhu (India). In addition, there were Muscle-tendon Strengthening Exercise of Dharma, Six Initial Approaches of Tiantai, Tibetan Vajrayana Vajra Boxing and other health preservation methods, all of which belong to the category of Buddhist health preservation.

What are the characteristics of Confucian health preservation school?

The purpose of Confucian health preservation is the mean and harmony view and self-cultivation. During the Warring States Period, Confucianism could only exist as one school of the "Nine Schools Among the Ten", and it was still in its infancy. In the Han Dynasty, in the time the Emperor Wu of Han, Dong Zhongshu put forward "venerating Confucianism". In the fifth year of the Emperor Wu of Han (136 BC), the court academician of Confucian classics was established, and consequently raised the status of Confucianism as an official school. With the rising status of Confucianism, Confucian health preservation began to gradually develop into an independent school. First of all, Dong Zhongshu combined health preservation with the doctrine of the mean, emphasizing nourishing qi and the mean and harmony view. Although *Huainanzi* written in the Western Han Dynasty tended to "oust Confucianism with Taoism", it gave full play to many reasonable parts of Confucianism and developed the Confucian theory of self-cultivation. Later, Xun Yue combined the Confucian theory of self-cultivation with qi, body and spirit, and expounded it theoretically, which made the Confucian theory of self-cultivation more closely related to human physiological and pathological changes and easier to popularize. By the Sui and Tang Dynasties, Confucian health preservation school had become very popular among officialdom and literati. Sun Simiao, a famous doctor and health preserver in the Tang Dynasty, is a figure of harmonious integration of Confucianism, Buddhism and Taoism. He especially listed a volume for health preservation in his book *Essential Recipes for Emergent Use Worth A Thousand Gold*, and named it "yangxing (self-cultivation)". In the Song Dynasty, with the supplement and exertion of Cheng Yi, Zhu Xi, Lu Jiuyuan, Wang Shouren and others, Confucian health preservation became more popular. In a word, the Confucian health preservation school was gradually formed after the Western Han Dynasty, when Confucian scholars linked the moral cultivation, moral consciousness and the mean and harmony view in Confucius and Mencius' theories with TCM health preservation methods. It has an inevitable connection with TCM health preservation, and also has its own characteristics.

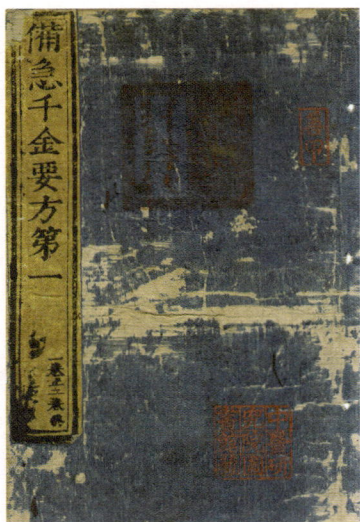

Essential Recipes for Emergent Use Worth A Thousand Gold (Bèi Jí Qiān Jīn Yào Fāng, 备急千金要方)

Preserved in China Academy of Chinese Medical Sciences (CACMS)

What are the ideological characteristics of doctor health preservation school?

Doctor health preservation school refers to the health preservation school using medicine and food as its main means. There are many fine branches in the doctor health preservation school. Those who mainly focus on health preservation with food are called food health preservation school, and those who mainly emphasize health preservation with medicine are called medicinal health preservation school. In medicinal health preservation school, it can be divided into spleen-regulating school, kidney-tonifying school, yin-nourishing, yang-strengthening school, etc. due to different medication habits.

How did the study of health preservation and healthcare develop and enrich during the Song, Jin, Yuan, Ming, and Qing Dynasties?

During the Song, Jin, and Yuan Dynasties, which were the later periods of feudal society in China, there was an ideological advocacy for the integration of Confucianism, Buddhism, and Taoism known as "Neo-Confucianism". Additionally, a philosophical school called "New Learning" emerged during this time. These schools had debates, mutual permeation, absorption, and development, which had certain influences on healthcare. After the Song Dynasty, the focus of health preservation and healthcare began to shift, and during the Ming and Qing Dynasties, a distinctive system of elderly health preservation was established. At the same time, the theory, variety, and methods of dietary health preservation continued to deepen and popularize. The rise of medical schools during the Jin and Yuan periods had a significant impact on TCM health preservation, especially the medical practitioners' approaches to health preservation. The period from the Song to the Ming and Qing Dynasties was the golden age of development for TCM health preservation. It was the period with the fastest development pace in the history of health preservation in ancient China, and many renowned health preservation experts emerged during this time. The characteristics of health preservation during this period are as follows.

First, the methods of health preservation and healthcare became more complete. The book *Taiping Holy Beneficence Prescription*, compiled by the imperial court of the Northern Song Dynasty, not only served as a comprehensive medical book with a complete system of principles, methods, prescriptions, and medicines but also contained many contents related to health preservation and healthcare. In the late Northern Song Dynasty, the government organized the compilation of *Shengji General Record*, a 200-volume, over 2 million-word collection, which included 66 categories such as internal medicine, external medicine, gynecology, pediatrics, ophthalmology, acupuncture and moxibustion, health preservation, and miscellaneous treatments. The content was rich, and the book provided a fairly detailed introduction to various methods of health preservation and healthcare.

Second, there was further development and enrichment in the health preservation and healthcare for the elderly. During the Jin and Yuan periods, academic debates led to a more refined understanding of health preservation theories and methods for the elderly. This was mainly reflected in the emphasis on mental regulation, dietary regulation, adherence to seasonal rhythms, attention to daily routines and care, and the use of appropriate medications.

Third, the negative tendencies in medicinal health preservation were corrected. The undesirable trend of using minerals and stones as medicines gradually received correction, bringing medicinal health preservation back on the right track.

Fourth, there was an abundance and popularization of dietary health preservation methods. With continuous accumulation of practical experience, there have been new developments in the theory and methods of dietary therapy and health preservation, leading to significant achievements.

Fifth, the "Four Great Masters" of the Jin and Yuan Dynasties had a significant influence on the study of health preservation. They were not only clinicians and theorists but also experts in health preservation. They played a crucial role in innovating and developing theories of health preservation. Among them, Liu Wansu emphasized the importance of cultivating vital energy (qi) for health preservation, Zhang Zihe advocated dispelling pathogenic factors and supporting the righteous, Li Dongyuan focused on regulating the spleen and stomach, and Zhu Danxi emphasized the nourishment of yin energy.

How did the study of health preservation revive and develop in modern times?

After the establishment of the People's Republic of China, the government began to pay attention to TCM health preservation industry. Corresponding institutions were established, and the number of books and papers on health preservation increased. Health preservation practices gradually became popular. By the mid-1950s, as economic and cultural development gradually improved, the TCM health preservation industry began to recover. Due to limited financial and material resources during this period, the focus of TCM work was on treating common and prevalent diseases that harm the health of the working people. Therefore, qigong health preservation, which was inexpensive and easy to popularize, emerged first. In July 1957, the Shanghai Qigong Rehabilitation Institute was established, marking a new stage in the development of qigong health preservation in China. After its establishment, the institute carried out notable qigong health preservation projects and conducted research on the relationship between qigong and meridians, as well as the detection and confirmation of meridians. During this period, a large number of TCM books were published, and the popularity of Western medicine in China promoted the development of TCM health preservation research.

In the late 1970s, the focus of the Party and the government shifted to economic development, with reform and opening-up becoming the basic national policy and the fundamental ideology for socialist construction in China. The Party and the government respected and valued science, and the era of science arrived, bringing springtime to TCM health preservation studies. Additionally, rapid developments in international geriatric medicine and the obvious trend of population aging provided momentum and opportunities for TCM health preservation studies. In June 1980, the Yue Meizhong Academic Experience Research Office was established at the Xiyuan Hospital of CACMS (China Academy of Chinese Medical Sciences), initiating research on TCM geriatrics and anti-aging medicine. Several papers were published, such as "Overview of Longevity Plants with Tonifying Effects" and "Overview of Anti-aging Animal Drugs", the latter of which was also translated into Japanese and published in Japan. Since the 1980s, ancient health preservation texts have been compiled and published, and research monographs by contemporary scholars have continued to emerge, greatly promoting the development of TCM health preservation studies during this period. In April 1988, the first session of Chinese Rehabilitation, Recuperation, and Health Preservation Academic Symposium was held in Qingdao, Shandong Province. More than 120 experts in rehabilitation, recuperation, and health preservation, including Xue Xiaoqin, Wang Fengqi, Wang Yuxue, and Sun Guangrong, gathered to exchange research achievements in health preservation studies.

In recent years, with the shift in medical models, the focus of medical scientific research has gradually shifted from clinical medicine to preventive medicine and rehabilitation medicine. Traditional health preservation and healthcare have experienced rapid development and a flourishing situation. In summary, there have been several main aspects: remarkable achievements in preventive healthcare, the establishment of research institutions for health preservation and healthcare, continuous progress in theoretical research, the promotion of social health education, innovations in health preservation education, and active academic exchange activities. The continuous development of TCM health preservation studies will make greater contributions to the health and longevity of the Chinese and people around the world.

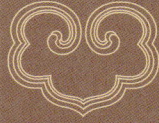

Chapter 2

Fundamentals of TCM

Health Preservation

Section 1
Tiannian

What is the natural life span?

Natural life span means the interval between the first breath and the last breath without any unexpected shortening of life. In ancient Chinese literature, natural life is often called "tiannian".

What is the natural life span that human beings should enjoy?

Basic Questions–Shanggu Tianzhen Lun pointed out that "live to an expected longevity and die after 100 years old"; *Miraculous Pivot–Tiannian* also said that "people die at the age of 100"; scholars in the Han Dynasty also said that "the different life spans caused by different physical strength are divided by 100 years old". *Laozi* puts forward that "the ultimate life span of human is 120 years old"; *The Book of History–Hongfan* recorded that "the natural life span is 120 years old". It can be seen that ancient Chinese doctors and scholars recognized the limit of human's "tiannian" as around 100 to 120 years old.

What is the boundary of aging?

Everyone has to go through such a life course as birth, development, growth, aging and death. Aging is a stage of life course. When does this stage start?

Miraculous Pivot–Tiannian recorded: "When a human turns ten years old, the five zang viscera become stable, and the blood and qi are unobstructed. The qi is going downward, so he tends to walk...At the age of forty, the five viscera and the twelve meridians are all in their prime and functioning harmoniously. The intercellular spaces begin to loosen, signs of prosperity and glory decline, and gray hairs start to appear. With stability and without disturbance, one prefers sitting calmly. The complexion begins to fade, and the hair is grizzled. He reaches his peak of life and stops developing, so he tends to sit. When he turns fifty years old, the liver qi begins to decline, and the liver lobes become thin. The bile begins to decrease, and he starts to lose his sight. When he turns sixty years old, the heart qi begins to decline. Therefore, he suffers from worries and sorrows. The blood and qi become sluggish, so he tends to lie down. When he turns seventy years old, the liver qi is deficient, and the skin is withered. At the age of eighty, lung qi weakens and the ethereal soul starts to detach, hence speech becomes prone to errors. When he turns ninety years old, the kidney qi is scorched, and the four zang viscera and meridians are empty. At the age of 100, all the five zang viscera are deficient..." It divide the human lifespan into units of ten years. It is considered that by the age of forty, although the body development is in its heyday, the signs of aging begin to emerge. *Basic Questions–Shanggu Tianzhen Lun* said: "When a woman turns seven years old, her kidney qi is prosperous. She starts to grow permanent teeth, and her hair grows fast. When she turns fourteen years old, her tiangui arrives, her conception vessel is unobstructed, and the qi and blood in her thoroughfare vessel are abundant. So the menstruation comes in time, and she is fertile. When she turns twenty-one years old, the kidney qi is balanced, so the permanent teeth are fully grown. When she turns twenty-eight years old, her tendons and bones are strong, and her hair is fully grown. Her body is also full of power. When she turns thirty-five years old, the vessel of yangming declines. Consequently, her complexion starts to look withered, and her hair begins to fall off. When she turns forty-two years old, the three yang vessels decline on the upper part of the body, the face is withered, and the hair begins to turn white. At the age of forty-nine, the conception vessel becomes deficient, the taichong meridian weakens and diminishes, the tiangui (heavenly essence) is exhausted, and the didao (reproductive system) is blocked. As a result, the physical body deteriorates and one becomes unable to have children. When a man turns eight years old, his kidney is solid. He starts to grow permanent teeth, and his hair grows fast. When he turns sixteen years old, the kidney qi is abundant, and his tiangui arrives. The essence is overflowing, and yin and yang are harmonious, so he is fertile. When he turns twenty-four years old, the kidney qi is balanced. His tendons and bones are strong and powerful, and the permanent teeth are fully grown. When he turns thirty-two years old, the muscles and tendons are bulging, and the bones are filled with marrow. When he turns forty years old, the kidney qi fails, the hair falls and the teeth are haggard. When he turns forty-eight years old, yang qi is exhausted on the top, the face is withered, and the hair begins to turn white. When he turns to fifty-six, the liver qi is exhausted, and the tendons are rigid. When he turns sixty-four years old, his tiangui is depleted, and there is little essence. The kidney is failing, and the body is reaching to its extreme. His teeth and hair all fall out." It is considered that men and women have different laws of growth and development. Women and men start to transfer from prosperity to descent at thirty-five and forty, respectively. It is obvious that the growth cycle of women is seven years, and that of men is eight years. Moreover, the time of life from prosperity to descent is 49 years in women, and 64 years in men. It can be seen that men have a whole more growth cycle than women. Therefore, women not only mature earlier, but also age earlier than men. In ancient Chinese literature, there are other sayings about the boundary of "old": "seventy years old is old", "eighty years old is old" (*Shuowen Jiezi*), "people over fifty are old" (*Miraculous Pivot*), etc. Summarizing various viewpoints, we can basically conclude that TCM regards forty to fifty years old as the period when the human body turns from prosperity to descent.

However, the process of aging is gradual, and everyone begins to age at different ages. Therefore, it is difficult to divide the boundaries of aging completely from age.

What are the morphological characteristics of aging?

What changes do people have in their appearance when they reach the aging period? *Basic Questions–Maiyao Jingwei Lun* pointed out: "Five zang viscera are the origin of a strong body. The head is the storage of essence and brightness. When the head is lowered and the gaze is unfocused, the spirit will decline. The back is the storage of the five zang viscera. If the back is bent and shoulders are drooping, the viscera will be damaged. The waist is the storage of kidney qi. If the waist can't be rotated, the kidney qi will be worn out. Knees are the storage of tendons and ligaments. If the knees can't bend and stretch, and one should bend the body and use aids when walking, the function of tendons and ligaments will decline. Bones are the storage of marrow. If one can't stand for a long time, and tremors and sways when walking, the function of bones will be exhausted." It vividly described various aging postures caused by hypofunction of viscera.

Acquisition of Knowledge through Profound Study–Theory of Health Preservation said: "Dizziness, abnormal eye scretion, itchy skin, frequent urination, runny nose, tooth loss, excessive saliva, little sleep, weakness of lower limbs, deafness, forgetfulness, vertigo, dry skin, dirty face, alopecia, dim eyesight, sedentary dozing, feeling cold before being exposed to wind, easiness to be hungry after eating, and easiness to laugh into tears are all manifestations of aging." It comprehensively summarized all kinds of manifestations when people begin to age.

Specifically, the appearance characteristics of aging include: whitening and shedding of hair; flabby and wrinkled skin, and muscle atrophy; the appearance of senile plaque; bone degeneration and tooth loss; changes in body structure, etc.

Section 2
Aging

What is the definition of aging?

What is aging? Scholars at home and abroad have many definitions of it. However, there has been no recognized definition of aging so far. In terms of the meaning of the word, there are aging and senescence in English. The latter is usually used to indicate the changes when the functions of animals are obviously declining in the late stage, while the word aging is used in the process of hypofunction. Others think that aging indicates gaining age or growing old in both the early and late stages of life. Therefore, the change that starts from puberty is called aging. However, in real life, the two are often used interchangeably.

What is the cause of aging in TCM?

Basic Questions–Shanggu Tianzhen Lun said: "I heard that people in ancient times can live to be more than 100 years old, and there are no signs of aging shown in their movements; nowadays, the movements of people are weak when they are only half a hundred years old. Is this caused by the difference of times? Or is it because today's people can't master health preservation?" This is a record of Huangdi asking Qi Bo why people at that time could not all live to a hundred as people in ancient times but instead started to age when they were over fifty. This question aroused the interest of TCM practitioners in the past dynasties, and they discussed the causes of aging from many aspects, which can be roughly classified into the following categories: irregular life, uncontrolled mood, differences in endowments and constitutions, geographical environment and climatic conditions.

How does irregular life lead to aging?

Regular and temperate life is of great significance to prevent and resist the occurrence of diseases and obtain health and longevity. *Basic Questions–Shanggu Tianzhen Lun* clearly pointed out: "Abide by the law of yin and yang, harmonize with appropriate ways of health preservation, eat and drink temperately, live a regular life, and avoid overwork and excessive sexual intercourse. In this way, the harmony of body and spirit can be achieved, and people can live to an expected longevity and die after a hundred years old." On the contrary, if violating the law of life for a long time, "people who take wine as soup, have sexual intercourse drunk, use up the essence and genuine qi for desire, are incapable of self-control and spirit-control, violate the law of life for a brief moment of joy, and live without temperance, will face their decline of life after fifty years old". That is to say, if people drink too much, the source of qi and blood will be damaged; if people have sexual intercourse drunk, the root of essence will be hurt; if people live without temperance, the body and qi will be shaken; if people are incapable of self-control for a brief moment of joy, the primordial genuine qi will be consumed. This practice of "taking the recklessness as the norm" leads to the "decline of life after fifty years old".

What aspects does irregular life include?

First, improper diet. As we all know, the life activities of the human body are mainly maintained by continuous intake of nutrients from the diet. The growth, reproduction and longevity of the human body are closely related to the intake of nutrition. An intemperate diet will lead to diseases and accelerate aging.

Second, excessive drinking. TCM believes that moderate drinking is acceptable, and that excessive drinking will cause damage to the body. *Miraculous Pivot–Discussion on Courage* pointed out that "liquor is the essence of water and grains, as well as the liquid of ripe grain, and its qi is fierce. When it enters the stomach, the stomach distends. And the adverse rising qi fills the chest, the liver qi is floated and feeble, and the gall bladder qi is obstructed". *Key to Diet* also pointed out: "It is better to drink less. Drinking excessively hurts the body and life span, changes people's personalities, which is especially poisonous. Excessive drinking is the source of death." Therefore, *Huangdi Neijing* regarded "taking wine as soup" as the reason for "declining after fifty years old".

Third, abnormal labor and rest. Moderate labor exercise and reasonable rest are important conditions tokeephuman body energetic, healthy and long-lived, and abnormal labor and rest is one of the factors affecting health and leading to premature aging. Therefore, *Huangdi Neijing* emphasizes "keeping the body labored but not tired", and *Basic Questions–Xuanming Wuqi* clearly put forward the viewpoint that "excessive use of eyes will hurt blood, long-time sitting will hurt muscles, long-time standing will hurt bones, long-time walking will hurt tendons and ligaments, and staying in bed for a long time will hurt qi", in which "long-time sitting" and "staying in bed for a long time" mean excessive resting; "long-time standing", "long-time walking", and "excessive use of eyes" mean excessive working. Both are harmful to health. Therefore, *Records of Cultivating Nature and Prolonging Life* pointed out that "the method of prolonging life only lies in not hurting the body...don't work either too hard, nor too relaxed..."

Fourth, excessive sexual intercourse. Appropriate sexual life is instinctive, natural, and wanton indulgence is the cause of premature aging and early death. *Basic Questions–Shanggu Tianzhen Lun* pointed out that "have sexual intercourse drunk, use up the essence and genuine qi for desire...will face their decline of life after fifty years old", which shows that excessive sexual intercourse will consume the important material basis of human life activities—essence. The deficiency of kidney essence leads to aging. TCM experts suggest that "those who are good at health preservation must conserve their essence".

What aspects does improper diet include?

Intemperate diet includes over-hunger, over-fullness, partiality for a particular kind of food, overly cold or overly hot diet.

What is over-hunger?

Over-hunger means insufficient food intake. The needs of normal life activities of human body cannot be met, and the source of qi and blood is insufficient, which can lead to premature aging over time. *Miraculous Pivot–Five Flavors* pointed out that "if the food is not taken, the qi will decline in half a day, and it will be less in one day".

What is over-fullness?

Over-fullness means eating too much, which is an important factor that damages human health and leads to aging. There is a saying in *Basic Questions–Discussion on Bi* that "if the diet amount is doubled, the intestines and stomach will be injured". It means that if you eat too much and the food intake exceeds the bearing capacity of the intestines and stomach, the spleen and stomach will be damaged, weakening its function of digesting, transporting and transforming the subtle essence of food and drink, and damaging the health of the body. Sun Simiao's *A Supplement to Recipes Worth A Thousand Gold* also said that "eating fully at night will cost a day of life", warning people not to eat too much, especially for dinner. In the Ming Dynasty, Ao Ying pointed out the harm of over-fullness in more detail in *Verbosity of Donggu*: "People who eat a lot have five hidden troubles: first, frequent defecation; second, frequent urination; third, troubled sleep; fourth, overweight; fifth, indigestion." Modern medicine believes that over-fullness will increase the burden on the gastrointestinal tract and cause indigestion, and it will lead to the concentration of blood in the gastrointestinal tract, which will cause ischemia of important organs, such as heart and brain, resulting in listlessness and even cardiovascular and cerebrovascular diseases. If people stay over-full for a long time and the food intake exceeds the needs of the body, the food will become fat stored in the body, which will lead to obesity, thus inducing a series of diseases that affect the life span.

What are the disadvantages of partiality for a particular kind of food?

Dietetic preference is the cause of disease and aging. *Basic Questions–Wuzang Shengcheng* said: "Overeating salty food results in blood coagulation and facial color change; overeating bitter food makes skin dry and haggard, and makes hair fall off; overeating pungent food makes the tendons tight and the nails dry; overeating sour food makes the thick muscles and lips shrink; overeating sweet food results in pain in the bones and hair loss. This is the damage caused by partiality of five flavors. Therefore, the heart wants bitter taste, the lung wants pungent taste, the liver wants sour taste, the spleen wants sweet taste, and the kidney wants salty taste. This is the corresponding relationship between the five flavors and the qi of the five viscera." It pointed out a series of pathological changes caused by the partial excess-deficiency of organs due to the partial preference for five flavors, and *Basic Questions–Zhizhenyao Dalun* also acknowledged the harm caused by the long-term partial excess of five flavors: "The long-term use of medicinals or food of the same flavor will result in the partial excess of qi, and the long-term excess of qi will lead to premature deaths." It shows that the long-term partial excess of five flavors can lead to premature aging and premature deaths. On this basis, *Basic Questions* also expounded the pathological changes caused by eating greasy and sweet food: "There is a disease that causes dry mouth...it is called spleen fever...it is caused by greasy and sweet food. People with this disease must have eaten greasy and sweet food very often. Greasy food can cause internal heat, and sweet food can result in distention" (*Basic Questions–Qibing Lun*). "Overeating greasy and sweet food will lead to *ding* (deep-rooted sore)" (*Basic Questions–Shengqi Tongtian Lun*).

What is the malpractice of overly cold or overly cold diet?

Having either an overly cold or overly cold diet can do harm to the body, which is also discussed in the *Huangdi Neijing*, such as "the excessive cold and heat of food and drink is harmful to the six fu viscera" (*Basic Questions–Yinyang Yingxiang Dalun*), and "drinking cold drinks when a person is attcked by cold pathogen hurts the lung" (*Miraculous Pivot–Xieqi Zangfu Bingxing*). Therefore, *Miraculous Pivot–Shi Zhuan* pointed out that "in terms of food and drink, they should be neither too hot nor too cold".

How does emotional disorder lead to aging?

According to TCM, mental activity is the governor of visceral activities. Only when people's emotional activities are smooth can visceral functions be balanced and coordinated and keep healthy. If an emotional disorder occurs, it will lead to various pathological changes. According to TCM theory, each viscus has its own emotional activity. *Basic Questions–Yinyang Yingxiang Dalun* said that "the five zang viscera develop five qi as joy, anger, sorrow, worry, and fear". The heart matches joy, the liver matches anger, the spleen matches sorrow, the lung matches worry and the kidney matches fear. Under normal circumstances, this is the normal mental and emotional activity of the human body. If the seven emotions are overwhelming or appear too urgently, they can become pathogenic factors and cause the disorder of qi activity in the human body. *Basic Questions–Jutong Lun* said: "I know that all diseases are caused by the changes of qi. Rage leads to qi ascending, excessive joy leads to qi loose, sadness leads to qi elimination, fear leads to qi sinking...fright leads to qi turbulence...and pensiveness leads to qi knotting." It shows that when the seven emotions are getting extreme, which exceeds the psychological and physiological adjustment ability of the body, it will result in disharmony between qi and blood, imbalance of yin and yang, and disorder of visceral function, leading to premature aging.

What is the relationship among natural endowment, constitution and aging?

TCM has long recognized that people's life span is related to their natural endowment and constitution. The so-called natural endowment mainly refers to genetic factors, while the constitution is the relatively stable inherent characteristic of function and form of the human body on the basis of heredity and acquisition. *Miraculous Pivot–Yinyang Ershiwu Ren* pointed out: "Fire-shaped people...mostly don't live long and may suddenly die." The reason they "don't live long" is probably influenced by inferior genetic elements in their constitutions. *Miraculous Pivot–Tiannian* recorded: "Huangdi asked: at the beginning of the human life, what builds its foundation? What builds its external defence? Qi Bo said: take the mother as the foundation and the father as the defence." Wang Chong pointed out more clearly in the *Discussion of Balance–Qishou*: "This refers to the different amount of qi that people are endowed with...If a person is endowed with more qi, his constitution will be strong, and he will have a long life. If a person is endowed with less qi, his constitution will be weak, and his life will be short."

What effects do climatic conditions and geographical environment have on aging?

People's life span is closely related to climatic conditions and geographical environment. When the wind, cold, summer heat, dampness, dryness and fire in nature turn abnormal, they will become the "six climatic exopathogens" that often lead to diseases in the human body. *Miraculous Pivot–Baibing Shisheng* said: "All kinds of diseases are caused by the changes of wind, cold, summer heat, dampness, dryness and fire." We should "timely avoid those pathogens". According to the different climate changes in spring, summer, autumn and winter, it also put forward "cultivating yang in spring and summer" and "nourishing yin in autumn and winter".

The influence of geographical environment on human life span is also discussed in *Huangdi Neijing*. In *Basic Questions–Wuchangzheng Dalun*, it is stated that "people living in the higher place have a long life span, while those living in the lower place have a short life span". Higher place refers to alpine areas with fresh air and cold climate; lower place refersto hot and humid low-lying areas. Because "the climate in the higher place is cold", the plants grow more slowly, and the growth period is long, so the life span is long; "the climate in the lower place is hot", so the plants grow faster and have a relatively short life span.

Section 3
Delaying Aging

What is the principle of delaying aging in TCM?

Prevent the disease before its onset and start health preservation before aging. The idea of preventing the disease before its onset is one of the important theories of TCM. *Basic Questions–Siqi Tiaoshen Dalun* pointed out: "Therefore, the sage does not wait for the disease to happen before treating it, but treats it before it happens. Just as he does not wait for the chaos to happen before containing it, but contains it before it happens. Treating the disease and containing the trouble before their occurrence are like digging a well when thirsty and making weapons in the war. Isn't it too late?" This idea of "preventive treatment of disease" is of great guiding significance for us to preserve our health and resist aging. Zhang Zhongjing inherited the academic thought of the *Huangdi Neijing*, and put forward the viewpoint of "cultivation and prevention", He thought that people should adjust the diet internally, practice daoyin and exhalation-inhalation, and not have excessive sexual intercourse, in order to nourish the primordial qi; they should also avoid cold and summer heat externally, conform to the four seasons, and be cautious of wind exopathogen. In this way, a life span of a hundred years can be achieved.

Broadly speaking, all methods of health preservation and preventing aging in TCM are aimed at preventing diseases, preserving health and prolonging life. For example, in terms of daily life adjustment, *Huangdi Neijing* emphasizes that "pathogens" such as "wind, rain, cold and summer heat" should be "timely avoided"; in terms of food hygiene, Zhang Zhongjing specially established *Eating Taboos of Animals, Fish and Insects* in *Treatise on Cold Damage* to emphasize the prevention of food poisoning. Sun Simiao recorded the use of animal liver to prevent nyctalopia in his works, as well as preventing endemic goiter with the thyroid gland of the sheep and seaweed. *Basic Questions–Cifa Lun* said that "the acupuncture technique has the significance of preserving the spiritual qi and recuperating the genuine primordial qi, and it also has the function of cultivating the genuine qi. Therefore, it does more than simply treating the diseases", which is the first of its kind for later generations to preserve health by acupuncture or moxibustion [such as moxibustion at Zúsānlǐ (ST36), Sānyīnjiāo (SP6), Qìhǎi (CV6), Guānyuán (CV4), Zhōngwǎn (CV12) and other acupoints]. Therefore, the guiding ideology of TCM health preservation should be to start health preservation before aging.

As we all know, the whole process of human life can be divided into several stages: birth, growth, strength, aging and death. Providing for the aged should not be implemented when entering the aging stage. TCM health preservation should not only be aimed at the elderly, but also at the young and the adult. Specifically, it should include fertilization, pregnancy, childbirth, nursing, raising the young, providing for the aged, etc. TCM has a large amount of experience and theories on this, such as attaching importance to eugenics, paying attention to prenatal education, caring for children's health and emphasizing middle-aged health prevention. It can be said that only by paying attention to raising the young and providing for the aged, can we get twice the result with half the effort.

What are the methods of delaying aging in TCM?

Roughly speaking, it includes three aspects: first, daily recuperation and temperate life; second, self-exercise and perseverance; third, combination of medicine and diet, and coordination of acupuncture and moxibustion.

What are the general aspects of daily recuperation?

Following the law of life, and paying attention to the aftercare in daily life, such as diet, lifestyle, sleep, labor and spirit, play an important role in delaying aging. TCM health preservation emphasizes proper diet, appropriate lifestyle and pleasurable mood. In the long-term medical care practice, a set of effective health preservation methods has been formed, such as the four-season health preservation method, lifestyle health preservation method, dietetic health preservation method, sleep health preservation method and mental health preservation method.

What are the methods of self-exercise in TCM?

Self-exercise methods in TCM include qigong, daoyin, massage, etc. The so-called qigong in modern times originated from ancient daoyin, exhalation-inhalation and other exercise methods, and the key lies in body adjustment, heart adjustment and breath adjustment. Qigong in China has a long history and developed into various schools. In terms of forms, it can be divided into two categories: static exercise and dynamic exercise. Daoyin is also a unique body-strengthening and life-prolonging method formed in ancient China. Its main function is to "guide the qi to achieve harmony, and stretch the body to achieve softness", so that the human body is full of energy and the blood circulation is smooth. Some of the categories of daoyin is mainly to regulate respiration, while others are mainly to stretch the limbs, such as Wuqinxi, Baduanjin, Yijinjing, and Taijiquan. Health-preservation massage has a long history in China, and its main function is to dredge blood vessels, harmonize qi and blood, strengthen visceral functions, and dispel various pathogens. Its specific methods can be divided into head massage, whole body massage, acupoint massage and so on. The above-mentioned methods are unique ways of TCM health preservation, which can eliminate internal and external interference and set the patient in the best state of unity of the body and spirit, thus implementing self-regulation on the whole life process, stimulating and mobilizing the internal potential of the human body, eliminating diseases, preventing aging and prolonging life.For individuals, they don't need to master all the methods. As long as they choose one that is suitable for themselves, keep exercising and persevere, they are bound to benefit.

What are the other ways to delay aging?

Medicinal health preservation: From time to time, it can be seen in the literature of TCM that many medicinals and prescriptions have the functions of "invigorating qi and lightening the body", "preventing aging and increasing life span" and "prolonging life", all of which belong to the category of medicinal nourishment. In recent years, traditional anti-aging traditional Chinese medicinals and prescriptions, especially those with the effect of tonifying the kidney, invigorating the spleen and benefiting qi, and promoting blood circulation, etc., have been studied emphatically, and the anti-aging mechanism of traditional Chinese medicinals has been preliminarily revealed from the aspects of immunity, metabolism, the adjustment of the nervous system, endocrine and visceral functions, anti-infection and the adjustment of trace elements.

Dietetic health preservation: The ancient people thought that "medicine and food are homologous" and "medicinal supplement is no better than dietetic supplement". Zhang Zihe even put forward the viewpoint that "health preservation must be achieved through dietetic supplement". Dietetic therapy is the main form of dietetic supplement. The prescription of dietetic therapy is generally composed of food and medicinals. It takes the nature of medicine, and uses the taste of food. The food borrows the power of the medicinals, and the medicinals help strengthen the force of the food. They complement each other, improve the immunity of the body to varying degrees, enhance the physiological function of the body, and have the function of strengthening the body and prolonging life.

In addition, there are many effective, simple and practical methods of health preservation and preventing aging in TCM, such as acupuncture health care, health preservation moxibustion, umbilical compress therapy and medicated pillow therapy.

Section 4
Three Most Precious Treasures

What is the meaning of the "three treasures"?

The "three treasures" have many meanings. *Laozi* said: "I have three treasures, and I keep and cherish them. One is mercy, one is frugality, and another is daring not to be the first in the crowd." *Mencius–Jinxin Part Two* said: "The three treasures of the feudal lords: land, people, and political affairs." The so-called three treasures in Buddhism refer to Buddha, Dharma and monk. Taoism believes that essence, qi and spirit are the internal three treasures, while ears, eyes, nose and mouth are the external three treasures. The three treasures in TCM mainly refer to essence, qi and spirit. For a healthy person, these three are indispensable. The essence of health preservation lies in recuperating these three basic substances of human life activities.

What is the relationship between essence and life activities?

The body is the foundation of life. Essence is the substance that constitutes the body and aids its growth and development, and it is the original substance that constitutes life. *Basic Questions–Jingui Zhenyan Lun* said: "Essence is the foundation of the body." *Miraculous Pivot–Jueqi* pointed out: "When a man and a women have sexual intercourse to bring a new life into existence, the substance formed before the body is called the essence." *Miraculous Pivot–Meridians* also pointed out: "The beginning of the birth of a human is to form the essence first, and the essence develops into the brain marrow." They all show that the essence is the primitive substance of life. When the essence of men and women combines, embryos are formed in the mother's body, forming the body and bringing about life. This essence is endowed by parents and is innate, so it is called the innate essence. It has the function of reproduction, so it is called the foundation of reproduction.

The essence is not only the original substance that constitutes the body and produces life, but also the basic material that maintains life activities and promotes human growth and development. *A Must Read for Medical Practitioners* said: "Once the body is formed, the essence derived from food is supplied and enters the stomach. When the essence derived from food is sprinkled on the six fu viscera, the qi arrives. And when it is harmonized in the five zang viscera, the blood is produced. Therefore, the essence is what people live on." After birth, people constantly ingest food and drink from the outside world. Under the action of the spleen and stomach, they are transformed into the subtle essence of food and drink, which is distributed throughout the body, nourishing viscera, bones and muscles, supplementing brain marrow, promoting growth and development, and maintaining life activities, which is called acquired essence. The acquired essence is hidden in the kidney, and the kidney essence declines with age. From the beginning of infancy, the essence in the kidney is gradually filled, and the permanent teeth and hair start to grow; the essence in adolescence is thriving, the reproductive function is mature, the brain marrow is abundant, the mind is clear, the thinking is quick, the eyes are bright, the hearing is great, the muscles are strong, the hair is thick, and the body is husky; in the old age, the essence declines, resulting in exhaustion of tiangui, less essence in men, menopause in women, the decline of the body and infertility, hair falling and haggard teeth, withered face and bones, deafness and blindness, and attenuation of all aspects of functions. Therefore, the essence is closely related to the birth, growth, strength, aging and death of the human body, and it is the original substance to maintain endless life activities.

What is the relationship between qi and life activities?

Qi originally belonged to the category of philosophy, and ancient philosophers thought that everything in the universe was produced by the movement and change of qi. *Zhouyi–Xici* said: "The coordination of the heaven and earth created the world." When the concept of qi was introduced into the medical field, it was used to explain people's life activities. *Basic Questions–Baoming Quanxing Lun* pointed out: "The coordinated qi of the heaven and earth is called a human." TCM holds that human life activities are produced by the movement and change of qi, and the movement form of qi is nothing more than ascending, descending, exiting and entering. *Basic Questions–Liuweizhi Dalun* said: "If the function of exiting and entering is abolished, the spiritual mechanism will be destroyed; if the function of ascending and descending vanishes, the qi will be left alone in peril. Without exiting and entering, there will be no birth, growth, strength, aging and death; without ascending and descending, there will be no birth, growth, transformation, collection and storage. There is nothing that does not possess the properties of ascending, descending, exiting and entering, ascending and descending." From the beginning of life, qi ascends and descends all the time. The respiration, digestion, absorption, hearing and vision, and actions of the human body are all produced by the movement of qi. The ascending, descending, exiting and entering of qi is endless, and they cooperate with one another, so as to inhale the fresh air and exhale the turbidity, and ascend lucidity and descend turbidity. They continuously carry out metabolism and maintain life activities. Therefore, qi transformation is the characteristic of life's existence. Qi transformation is realized through the ascending, descending, exiting and entering movement of qi. Qi is intangible with quality, has strong mobility and is ubiquitous. Through the ascending, descending, exiting and entering movement, the power of life is generated, which stimulates the functional activities of maintaining viscera and tissues and continuously carries out qi transformation, thus generating life phenomena. Therefore, qi is the motive power of life activities.

What is the relationship between spirit and life activities?

Spirit can be divided into a broad sense and a narrow sense. Spirit in TCM not only refers to people's spiritual consciousness and thinking activities, but also summarizes complex life images, and is the master of all life activities. The existence of spirit is attached to the body and develops in accordance with the body, from nothing into something, and from weak to strong. The unity of the body and spirit is called a human. *Miraculous Pivot–Tiannian* said: "Once the blood and qi have been harmonized, the nutrient qi and defense qi have been unobstructed, the five zang viscera have been established, the spirit has been stored in the heart, and the soul and inferior spirit have been in position, a human being is completed." Spirit is the external manifestation of life activities, and dominates all life activities. Only when the spirit is preserved can all human life activities be manifested. Therefore, Li Dongyuan said in *Treatise on the Spleen and Stomach* that "accumulate qi to produce essence and accumulate essence to complete spirit". Only when the essence is abundant, the qi is sufficient, and the spirit is completed, can people live a long and healthy life. All the experts in health preservation in the past dynasties paid great attention to spirit cultivation, "those who have spirit will prosper, and those who don't will die", "the best way to preserve health is to cultivate the spirit, and secondly, to cultivate the body".

What is the relationship among the "three treasures"?

Essence is the foundation of producing spirit. Qi is the motive force of transforming essence. Spirit is the external manifestation of essence and qi, which resides in essence and qi and is the master of essence and qi. All three are indispensable and are the foundation of human life activities. Therefore, *Categorized Patterns with Clear-cut Treatments* pointed out that "the treasure of the human body is the essence, qi, and spirit. The spirit is born in qi, and the qi is born in essence. The essence can transform into qi, and the qi can transform into spirit. Therefore, the essence is the foundation of the body, the qi is the governor of spirit, and the body is the house of spirit".

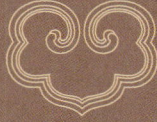

Chapter 3

Cultivating the Body

Section 1
Living A Regular Life

| Conforming to the rhythm of life

Why do people need to live a regular life?

From the movement changes of celestial bodies to the life activities of human bodies, there are inherent rhythms, and the life activities of human bodies cannot leave the rhythmic laws for a moment. TCM has long known this, and thinks that the qi and blood of human are affected by the sun, moon and stars. Periodic ups and downs occur due to the influence of the four seasons, so living a regular life should be noticed in health preservation to conform to the changes of yin and yang.

What should people do to live a regular life?

First of all, to live a regular life, people should conform to the rhythm of life, including daily rhythm, seasonal rhythm, five evolutive phases and six climatic factors and so on; second, they should maintain proper sleep; third, they should pay attention to physical care.

How does it conform to the yin and yang of the day?

Basic Questions–Shengqi Tongtian Lun said: "During the day, the body's yang qi mainly governs the surface of the body. In the early morning, the yang qi begins to be active and tends to go outward; at noon, the yang qi reaches its peak; when the sun sinks in the west, the yang qi gradually weakens and the pores begin to close. Therefore, at night, yang qi converges and defends on the inside. At this time, don't disturb bones and muscles, and don't approach the fog and dew. If people violate the law of yang qi in these three times of the day, their bodies will be sleepy and thin." It means that the yang qi is at its peak at noon in one day, and it declines in the evening. People should adapt to this change in their daily life, work at sunrise, and rest at sundown. Otherwise, the body will be easily damaged.

How does it conform to yin and yang of the four seasons?

According to TCM, people live in nature and are closely related to nature.

Only by adapting to the changes of the yin and yang in the four seasons can people be healthy. The rhythm of the four seasons is the law of birth in spring, growth in summer, harvest in autumn and storage in winter. *Basic Questions–Siqi Tiaoshen Dalun* said: "The change of yin and yang at four seasons is the foundation of all lives. Therefore, the wise men cultivate yang in spring and summer, and nourish yin in autumn and winter, in order to obey the fundamental law of life development. In this way, they can move and develop in the life process like all creatures. If this law is violated, the vitality will be attacked and genuine qi will be destroyed. Therefore, the change of yin and yang at four seasons is the beginning and end of all things and the foundation of life and death. If it is violated, disasters will take place. If it is obeyed, serious illness won't occur, which can be described as knowing the way of health preservation." It emphasizes that the change of yin and yang in four seasons has great influence on the human body, and people's health will be preserved if conforming to this law. If it is violated, various diseases will occur. Therefore, the general principles of "cultivating yang in spring and summer" and "nourishing yin in autumn and winter" were put forward. In terms of specific practices, it is advocated that people should "go to bed at night and get up early to walk casually in yard" in spring, "go to bed at night and get up early, and not avoid the long hours of sunshine" in summer, "go to bed early and get up as early as chickens" in autumn, and "go to bed early and get up late till the sun shines" in winter.

How does it adapt to the changes of the year?

Basic Questions–Liuyuan Zhengji Dalun said: "First of all, it is necessary to establish the stems and branches of the calendar, so as to understand the qi that domains the year, the five movements of metal, wood, water, fire and earth, and the transformation of six qi, such as cold, summer heat, dryness, dampness, wind, and fire. Then the changing law of nature can be discovered, and people can recuperate their bodies according to this law." It means that according to the theory of five element motions and six climate changes in TCM, the changing law of the climate each year and its impact on the human body can be calculated, and people can take targeted prevention and health-preserving measures accordingly. For example, when there is too much precipitation, the water and dampness are spreading, and the air becomes humid. The human body is vulnerable to dampness exopathogen, so moistureproof should be especially noticed in daily life. Food and drink (such as eating more pungent and warm foods) and medicinals (relatively more aromatic products) can be adopted to fight against dampness.

‖ Moderate labor and rest

What is labor and what is rest?

There is a dialectical unity relationship between labor and rest. They are opposite and coordinate with each other. Both of them are the physiological needs of the human body. According to TCM, labor includes physical overstrain, psychological overstrain and sexual overstrain. Rest means being easy and comfortable. Labor and rest are relative. Excessive fatigue will damage the body, and excessive comfort will also cause illness. People should both work and rest appropriately in their daily life.

Regular and reasonable physical and mental labor is conducive to promoting qi and blood circulation, exercising tendons and bones, enhancing metabolism, and strengthening thebrain and spirit. Some meaningful labor work can also edify sentiment and broaden the mind, so as to maintain vigorous energy and a delighted mood, strengthen the constitution and prevent diseases. However, labor must be moderate, especially for the elderly who are engaged in mental and physical labor. Overwork should be avoided. Otherwise, it will result in diseases.

However, people should not get too comfortable. TCM believes that "the body should not get too comfortable, otherwise the circulation of qi and blood will be stagnated, which will easily result in illnesses". In daily life, if people don't take part in physical exercise like a parasite whose four limbs do not toil, are well-fed all day long, and care about nothing, the circulation of qi and blood will be stagnated, the bones and muscles will be fragile, and the digestive function of spleen and stomach will decrease, leading to loss of appetite, feeble body, decreased resistance and so on.

What are the hazards of overstrain?

TCM believes that people should not be engaged in too much labor, and excessive labor will cause internal injuries to the viscera. As stated in *Basic Questions –Xuanming Wuqi*, five types of damage caused by improper work and leisure, that is, "excessive use of eyes will hurt blood, staying in bed for a long time will hurt qi, long-time sitting will hurt muscles, long-time standing will hurt bones, and long-time walking will hurt tendons and ligament". The so-called "Five Exhaustions" are the five most common unhealthy habits in people's daily lives. They can cause harm to the five viscera of the human body, leading to diseases associated with overexertion. Hence, ancient people often said, "Accumulated exhaustion leads to illness" and "The Five Exhaustions are most likely to harm the body".

Hua Tuo, a famous doctor in the Eastern Han Dynasty in China, thought that "the human body needs constant exercise, but it must not be excessive. When the human body moves, the nutrients in food can be digested, and the blood vessels are unobstructed, so people will not get sick, just like when the door is opened and closed frequently, the door pivot does not rot" (*Book of Later Han Dynasty*), and thought that a certain amount of work or exercise was beneficial to the human body, which should not be excessive so as not to harm the body. Sun Simiao also pointed out that "it is difficult to live long if people don't know the method of nature cultivation. The way to cultivate one's nature is often to work moderately. Do not overwork beyond physical capacity" (*Essential Recipes for Emergent Use Worth A Thousand Gold*), which clearly pointed out that if people want to live long, they must master health preservation, and the focus of it lays in "often working moderately", which requires a little fatigue. The ancients thought that people who were too comfortable in life could not live long, just as stagnant water with rotten smell and cut down trees with insects.

Why should we advocate exercise for health preservation?

Master Lv's Spring and Autumn Annals said: "Running water will not stink, and the door shaft that often rotates will not rot, so is the shape and qi. If the shape is not moving, the essence will not flow, and qi will be depressed." *Introduction to Medicine* recorded: "Sitting upright all day long is the most important thing that leads to death. People only know that walking and standing for a long time hurt people, but they don't know that sitting for a long time hurts people especially." It can be seen that ancient health preservers were aware of the significance of exercise to life, and TCM believes that exercise can promote the circulation of qi and blood, dredge meridians and normalize functional activities of viscera, which is beneficial to prolonging life.

What are the sports for health preservation?

In the long-term practice of fighting against diseases and pursuing longevity, the ancient people summarized and invented many methods of strengthening the body with strong national color. For example, in the Spring and Autumn Period and the Warring States Period, people imitated the actions of animals and created Erqinxi (bears climbing and birds stretching); in the Western Han Dynasty, Sanqinxi (bears, birds and apes) came into being; Hua Tuo inherited the rule of "exhaling the old and inhaling the new like bears climbing and birds stretching" in *Zhuangzi* and created Wuqinxi applying exercise health preservation; in the Jin Dynasty, new exercises such as swallows flying, snake curling, rabbit startling and turtles swallowing; in the Tang Dynasty, there were Baduanjin and Shierduanjin; there was the "sitting exercise" in the Song Dynasty; in the Ming Dynasty, there was Taijiquan, Shaolin martial arts, etc.

Nowadays, there are many fitness programs suitable for human beings, including the following several methods. Traditional fitness methods: qigong, daoyin, health massage, martial arts and so on; modern exercise methods: including walking, running, swimming, driving, ball games, etc.; medical sports: such as specialized medical rehabilitation exercises for chronic obstructive pulmonary disease and hypertension; natural fitness methods: including sunbathing, cold water bathing, mineral spring bathing, forest therapy, air therapy and so on. When choosing the type of exercise, we should do it properly, start

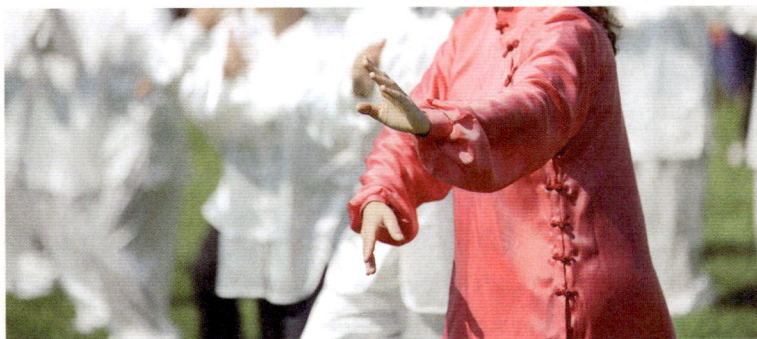

Taijiquan

early, persevere and combine dynamic and static according to the specific situation of individuals.

How to combine dynamic and quiescence?

Ancient health preservation experts advocated dynamic on the one hand and quiescence on the other, and emphasized the combination of dynamic and quiescence. Those who gave priority to quiescence were Laozi and Zhuangzi. Laozi thought that "quiescence is the master of restlessness" (*Tao Te Ching*), and strongly advocated "achieving empty and keeping quiet", that is, to eliminate distractions, stick to quiescence, and "maintain pure and simple nature and reduce selfish desires and distractions". Zhuangzi inherited Laozi's theories, and put forward that "by maintaining peace of mind, the body will naturally be healthy. Keep the heart clean and quiet, don't wear out the body, and don't drain the spirit. In this way, people can achieve longevity" (*Zhuangzi–Zaiyou*). It can be seen that Taoism, represented by Laozi and Zhuangzi, basically advocates "a quiet life of inaction" to keep in good health. *Master Lv's Spring and Autumn Annals* put forward the famous viewpoint that "running water will not stink, and the door shaft that often rotates will not rot", and advocated health preservation by keeping moving. In the time of Confucius, he put forward the viewpoint that "act in moderation and morality, and show joy and anger at the right time. In this way, the noble temperament will not be impaired", and advocated the combination of dynamic and quiescence (*Confucius's Words to Family*).

Ancient health preservation experts advocated that quiescence is aimed at cultivating the mind. They thought that if the heart was pure and less selfish, the spirit could be hidden inside, and the body could live outside at ease. The essence is to nourish the "body" by calming the "spirit". Therefore, many techniques of cultivating the mind with quiescence have been established. However, "quiescence" is only a special form of exercise, not absolute motionless. Laozi, Zhuangzi and others, while emphasizing quiescence, created dynamic fitness methods, such as daoyin and exhalation-inhalation. Therefore, the best health preservation method is the combination of dynamic and quiescence, and the combination of nourishing the body and spirit.

||| Proper sleep

What is sleep health preservation?

Sleep health preservation refers to a health preservation method that eliminates fatigue, regulates yin and yang and restores spirit through sleep. One-third of life is spent in sleep, and adequate and good sleep is an important factor in ensuring physical and mental health. The sleep that is beneficial to the human body must first be a good sleep.

What are the ways to have a good sleep?

First, the pure sleep method. Before going to bed, people should keep the body and mind quiet, with the mind cleared and with little desire. Don't think about problems 30 minutes before going to bed. It is best to do some activities to relax the brain tension, such as walking, listening to light music and opera, which are conducive to accelerating falling asleep. There is a saying by the ancients that "after Fu Weng was dismissed from his post, he snored as soon as he went to bed". It can be seen that if people want a good sleep, they should "rest the mind first, then the eyes", and they can fall asleep only when the mind is quiet and the spirit is calmed.

Second, the labor sleep method. Adding some proper physical activities during the day to make the body tired is conducive to sleep, such as walking before going to bed, exercising Baduanjin, etc. The ancients said that "after Xuanyuan finished swimming, he fell asleep against the wall", which shows that proper physical activity can help with sleep. But don't exercise strenuously before going to bed, just as the ancients said, "walking will make the body tired, and when the body is tired, people feel like to sleep."

Third, the diet sleep method. Some medicated diets and porridge which are beneficial to sleep can be properly selected to aid sleep. But eating too much before going to bed should be avoided, and do not drink stimulating drinks such as tea, wine or coffee before going to bed.

What is the sleep posture advocated by the ancients?

The ancients were also very particular about sleeping posture. *Xiyi Sleeping Tactics* advocates: when lying on the right side, bend the right leg; flex the right arm and support the head with the hand; stretch the left leg and place the hand between the thighs. If lying on the left side, the posture is contrary to what has been mentioned above.

Buddhism stipulated that people should lie on the right side, and named it "auspicious sleep". It is also scientifically reasonable, because man's heart is on the left side, and lying on the left side may oppress the heart.

How does "Zi Wu Liu Zhu" of TCM affect sleep?

The theory of Zi Wu Liu Zhu is a unique concept in TCM. Zi Wu refers to the twelve two-hour time periods in a day, while Liu Zhu means the flow and infusion. A day is divided into twelve two-hour period, namely Zi, Chou, Yin, Mao, Chen, Si, Wu, Wei, Shen, You, Xu and Hai, each time period corresponds to two hours in the present day, and each time period has different meridians "on duty". Lung meridian corresponds to Yinshi (the time of tiger); large intestine meridian corresponds to Maoshi; stomach meridian corresponds to Chenshi (the time of dragon); spleen meridian corresponds to Sishi (the time of snake); heart meridian corresponds to Wushi (the time of horse); small intestine meridian corresponds to Weishi (the time of goat); bladder meridian corresponds to Shenshi (the time of monkey); kidney meridian corresponds to Youshi (the time of chicken); pericardium meridian corresponds to Xushi (the time of dog); triple energizer meridian corresponds to Haishi (the time of pig); gallbladder meridian corresponds to Zishi (the time of rat), and liver meridian corresponds to Choushi (the time of ox)." The qi and blood in the human body also flow and circulate among the meridians in a certain rhythm. They have periods of abundance and decline, interconnect with each other, and maintain an orderly sequence. Taking the Zi time period as an example, which is from 11 pm to 1 am, the gallbladder meridian is "on duty" during this time. According to TCM theory, "The surplus qi of the liver flows into the gallbladder, gathering and forming essence". If one goes to bed before the Zi time period and wakes up in the morning, the mind will be clear, the complexion will be rosy, and there will be no dark circles. On the contrary, if one has a pale and dark complexion with dark circles around the eyes, it indicates imbalances. Therefore, it is recommended to prioritize sleep during the Zi time period and avoid staying up late or eating late-night snacks for better health.

IV Living environment

When did ancient TCM practitioners first know the relationship between the geographical living environment and life span?

Basic Questions–Wuchangzheng Dalun said: "Why are the growth, transformation, life span and death different in one state? Qi Bo said: it is caused by the difference of terrains. Places with high terrain are governed by yin qi, while places with low terrain are governed by yang qi. The climate in places with abundant yang is warm, and the growth and transformation of all lives often occur prior to four seasons; while the climate in places with abundant yin is cold, and all lives often occur later than four seasons. This is a geographical routine and affects the law of late and early growth and transformation. Huangdi asked: is there any difference in life span and death? Qi Bo said: places of high altitude is governed by yin qi, so the lives there can live long; places of low altitude is governed by yang qi, so the lives there die early. However, the difference in terrain is different to some extent. The difference in life span is small if the difference in terrain is small, and the difference in life span is big if the difference in terrain is big." It means that people living in high mountains with fresh air and cold climate live longer, while those living in low-lying areas with polluted air and hot climate live shorter. It can be seen that TCM recognized the relationship between the living environment and life span as early as more than 2, 000 years ago, so *Huangdi Neijing* put forward that health preservation should be "harmonious with yin and yang and content with the living environment".

How does geographical environment affect human health?

Master Lv's Spring and Autumn Annals recorded: "Where there is little water, there are many people with no hair on the head and goiter; where there is a lot of water, there are many people with swollen feet and people who can't walk because of foot diseases; where the water tastes sweet, there are many kind and beautiful people; where the water tastes spicy, there are many carbuncle sores and people with evil sores; where the water tastes bitter, there are many people with chicken breasts and curved backs." It means that people who have lived in the rain and dew for a long time are prone to hair loss and gall; people who have lived in places with well water for a long time often suffer from swollen feet and lame legs; people who have lived in the land of clear springs for a long time have beautiful looks; people who have lived in places with hot springs for a long time are prone to ding and furuncle; people who have lived in areas of barren alkali soil for a long time are prone to pigeon breasts, hunchbacks and other diseases. It can be seen that the living environment is very important to health.

What aspects of residence will have an impact on health preservation?

First, the orientation of the house. *House Classics* pointed out that if the windows face south, southeast or southwest, the indoor daylighting is good. Residential orientation affects not only daylighting, but also indoor ventilation. In most regions of China, it is reasonable for the residence to face south, which can make full use of the sun's illumination and air circulation, making the residence warm in winter and cool in summer.

Second, the residential address. The choice of living place belongs to one of the contents of "detecting fengshui", which was not a matter for doctors in the early days, but a matter for the yin-yang (geomancy) school. Doctors only put forward some principled suggestions for the needs of human health. For example, Sun Simiao has a section on "Choosing Land" in *A Supplement to Recipes Worth A Thousand Gold.* He thought that the deep mountain forest, quiet and delicate, is certainly a good environment for building houses, and emphasized that "a place with a good terrain is also good for living". In rural areas where conditions permit, houses should be built in places close to mountains and rivers. Because the house is by the mountain, trees in the mountains can keep out the wind, sand and cold in winter; in summer, dense trees can reduce sunlight radiation, absorb heat, adjust the temperature, reduce and eliminate noises, and keep the environment quiet. Also, clear running water can remove turbid air.

Third, landscaping. Beautifying the living environment is conducive to health and longevity. *Dixinshu* pointed out that residential areas should be widely planted with trees and bamboo around them, so as to make people feel fresh and vibrant. *Laolao Hengyan* advocated "planting dozens of flowers and trees in the courtyard, and not requiring precious and exotic breeds", as long as they bloom all the year round; "storing water in a big tank in front of the steps, and raising some goldfish", and "it doesn't hurt to do everything by yourself", which not only beautifies the environment and exercises the body, but also supports the body and mind. If conditions permit, people can plant trees and grass in front of and behind the house, making the pines luxuriant and the cypress verdant, all lush and living with shady grass. For urban residents living in modern cities, they should adjust measures to local conditions, and make full use of balconies and windowsills. Potted flowers and scandent plants can be selected, with vines creeping and flowers competing in a beauty contest, which can also detain the green.

How do people choose a living room?

The living room is the most important place for people's activities, and they spend almost half of their lifetime there. For the requirements of the living room, the ancients thought that the living room should not be too high or too low, but should be moderately spacious. *Tianyinzi* said that "the living room should have moderate yin and yang, and equal light and shade. The house should not be too high, otherwise there will be too much sunshine and brightness; the house should not be too low, otherwise there will be too much yin qi and darkness". From a modern point of view, the living room should have good sunshine, and the height of the living room should meet the requirements of daylighting and the natural circulation of air. The height of the room should be about 3 meters, and the room should be warm and comfortable, with sufficient light, good ventilation and without dampness. There is also another emphasis on the living room of the elderly. *Yanglao Fengqin Shu* pointed out that the living room where the elderly live must be elegant and clean, well-ventilated in summer and warm in winter; the bed for the elderly should be stable and lower than the bed used by ordinary people. The three sides of the bed should have bedrails, and the bedding and cushions on the bed must be flat and soft; if conditions permit, gauze curtains should be hung in summer above the bed and cloth curtains in winter, which can prevent mosquito bites and keep out the wind and cold.

How to beautify rooms for health preservation?

Beautiful and comfortable rooms have a good influence on people's psychology and physiology. There is no specific standard for beautifying rooms. The general principle is to decorate rooms according to their own tastes and hobbies. Room beautification should not be too luxurious. *Essential Recipes for Emergent Use Worth A Thousand Gold* said: "The living places should not be extravagant and gorgeous, making people greedy and insatiable, which is the source of disasters. The room should be simple, elegant and clean, without wind, rain, summer heat and dampness." It is thought that the settings inside the room do not need to be too gorgeous and extravagant. Extravagance can only increase people's greed for material desires and is the root of all harm. As long as the bedroom is light and elegant, simple and clean, it is the best shelter from the wind and rain and can provide protection against summer heat and dampness. In addition, according to the room size, personal hobbies, economic applicability, etc., placingpots of flowers, raising birds, feeding fish, self-decorating a few small bonsai, or hanging up a few famous calligraphy and paintings can cultivate people's nature and involve them in happiness. As for the placement of the bedroom furniture, it should be based on the principle of being neat, practical, harmonious, and convenient for rest and activities.

Section 2
Following the Law of Yin and Yang

| Health preservation in spring

What are the climatic characteristics of spring?

The *Huangdi Neijing* said: "The three months of spring are the period of sprouting and growing. The heaven and earth begin to generate [yang qi], and everything begins to flourish. In spring, it is desirable to sleep late at night, get up early in the morning, and take a walk in the yard. One should loosen up one's hairs and relax one's body to facilitate the development of one's emotions. The spring possesses the will to generate. After things have been generated, do not destroy them. One should assist things rather than taking them away; one should give awards rather than make punishment. This is according to the spring qi, and is the way of health cultivation. To live a lifestyle contrary to the spring will cause injuries to the liver and one will suffer a cold disease in the summer that follows."

The three months of spring begin at the Beginning of Spring and end at the Beginning of Summer. Spring is the season when everything grows. When spring returns to the earth, the ice and snow melt and yang rises. Everything recovers, and insects begin to move. The earth is full of vitality, and everything is thriving. Yang qi of the human body also goes with the flow, spreading upward and outward. However, the climate often changes in spring. For example, after suddenly getting warmer, the weather will turn cold again.

How do people cultivate the spirit in spring?

Everything blooms in spring, and spirit cultivation should be in line with the vitality of nature. The corresponding viscus of spring is the liver that controls conveyance and dispersion and has an aversion to depression. Therefore, in spring, people should keep an open mind and an optimistic mood, have no worries and refrain from getting angry. In the sunny spring, people should not stay at home all day long. Instead, they should go for an outing to visit the willows, mountains and rivers, watch flowers and springs, and cultivate their sentiments, so as to make themselves happy in spirit, comfortable in mood and integrate with nature.

How do people recuperate daily life in spring?

In spring, the climate gets warmer, and the activities of various systems of the human body are strengthened, which increases the load of various organs and produces the feeling of sleepiness that is called "spring drowsiness" by the folk. In order to adapt to this change, people should go to bed at night and get up early, loosen hair, stretch bodies and walk in the courtyard. At the same time, the climate is changeable in spring, and is easy to get cold or warm. Attention should be paid to preventing wind and cold, nourishing yang and gathering yin. In terms of clothing, "clothes that prevent the cold should not be taken off suddenly...prepare clothes that can be put on and take off according to the weather. Moreover, clothes should not be taken off a lot all of a sudden but one by one". There is a folk saying that "wear more clothes in spring and less in autumn", which is indeed a talk of experience. Spring is also a season suitable for physical exercise. The spring is bright, the air is fresh, and everything is colorful and full of vitality. If people can "get up upon hearing the rooster crow for physical exercise", it will help the human body to expel the stale and imbibe the fresh, practice the qi, preserve the essence and keep fit. This not only cultivates the mind but also exercises the body.

How do people recuperate by diet in spring?

When yang qi rises in spring, the human body function is also in full swing. The diet should be pungent, sweet and warm. The pungent and sweet food belongs to yang, which can help with the initial growth of spring yang. Warm food is conducive to protecting yang, and sour and greasy food should be avoided. The liver is active in spring, and the hyperactive liver wood can restrict the spleen earth. Therefore, *Essential Recipes for Emergent Use Worth A Thousand Gold* pointed out that the spring diet should "reduce acid and increase sweetness to nourish spleen qi", and *Shesheng Xiaoxi Lun* said "don't drink too much, and don't eat too much rice and cakes, which will hurt the spleen and stomach and do harm to digestion".

How do people take medications for health preservation in spring?

In spring, yang qi is growing, and everything is reviving. It is easy for various toxic exopathogens to spread, such as cold, influenza, upper respiratory tract inflammation, epidemic cerebrospinal meningitis, and measles. In addition to active treatment, attention should be paid to air disinfection. Indoor fumigation with wormwood leaf and vinegar can prevent influenza. At the same time, oral administration of traditional Chinese medicinals such as Banlangen (Isatidis Radix), Guanzhong (Dryopteridis Crassirhizomatis Rhizoma), Gancao (Glycyrrhizae Radix et Rhizoma), etc., can play a preventive role. Spring is also the onset period of many chronic diseases, such as cardiovascular and cerebrovascular diseases, and allergic asthma. In addition to treatment, TCM also advocates putting prevention first. For example, *A Supplement to Recipes Worth A Thousand Gold* pointed out that "three or five doses of Xiaoxuming Decoction for ordinary people in spring and one dose of each tonic powders" can strengthen the body and prevent diseases. *Shoushi Midian* also said that "in March, picking peach blossoms, soaking them in wine and then drinking the wine can eliminate all diseases and benefit complexion". These are all useful health preservation methods.

‖ Health preservation in summer

What are the climatic characteristics of summer?

Huangdi Neijing said: "The three months of summer are the period of prosperity and blossom. Qi of the heavens and that of the earth begin to interact with each other, which causes ten thousand things to blossom and bear fruits. In summer, it is desirable to sleep late at night and get up early in the morning, to have no dislike of sunlight. One should not be angry in summer, and keep himself spiritual just in accordance with the beautiful blossom [in the natural world]. One should let qi move outward through perspiration as if in love with the outside world. This is the good lifestyle to maintain in response to the summer. To live a lifestyle contrary to the summer will cause harm to the heart and one will suffer yin malaria in the autumn that follows."

The three months of summer begin at the Beginning of Summer and end at the Beginning of Autumn. Summer is a prosperous and beautiful season for all lives. The yang qi of the heaven drops, and the heat of the earth steams. Because of the mixing of the yang qi from upper heaven and the yin qi from lower earth, all lives begin to bear fruit. In summer, the climate is hot, and the yang qi of the human body is also very exuberant.

How do people cultivate the spirit in summer?

In summer, when the summer heat is in season, the climate is hot, and the corresponding viscus is the liver. Yang is outward, and the yin is concealed inside. In regard of spirit cultivation, attention should be paid to keeping a calm, peaceful and joyful mood, and avoiding getting angry. For example, *Shesheng Xiaoxi Lun* said: "It is better to adjust the breath and keep calm. In this way, even when the weather is hot, the heat in one's heart is reduced. Do not add heat to heat, otherwise more heat will be generated." In order to adapt to the hot weather in summer, we can take measures to cool off and avoid summer heat. In a word, the key point of spirit cultivation in summer is to try to be extroverted and open-minded.

How do people recuperate daily life in summer?

The climate is hot in summer. The daytime is longer and the nighttime is shorter. People are suggested to go to bed late and get up early, and take a proper nap to preserve energy. Summer heat prevails in summer. Therefore, it is advisable to prevent exposure to sunshine, lower room temperature, pay attention to indoor ventilation, and avoid heatstroke. In addition, people should avoid sleeping in the wind and being attacked by wind during sleep. Particularly "the elderly should be carefully protected, and should not cool off under the eaves, in the corridors, in the alleys and beside the broken windows. In these places, though it is cool, the elderly are apt to be attacked by wind. It is suitable for the elderly to obtain naturally coolness in the well-ventilated and clean rooms, the water pavilion, under the shade of trees, and in the neat and broad spaces" (*Shesheng Xiaoxi Lun*). Clothes should be light-colored, loose, breathable and heat-dissipating. In summer, people usually sweat a lot. Therefore, people should take a bath often, and wash and change clothes frequently. Physical exercises should not be ignored in summer. People is advised to choose to go to parks, lakeside and trees in the early morning or evening. The main exercises are those less energetic, such as walking, jogging, Taijiquan, qigong, swimming and so on.

How do people recuperate by diet in summer?

The climate is hot in summer, which corresponds to the heart fire. *Synopsis of Golden Chamber* pointed out that "people should not eat food that corresponds to the heart in summer". That is, according to the viewpoint of "supplementing the heart with heart" in TCM visceral dietetic therapy, it is considered that the heart is strong in summer and should not be supplemented more. *Key to Diet* recorded that "the qi in summer is hot, eating beans is advised to cool it down", advocating adapting to the changes of the four seasons with cold, hot, dry and damp food. *Book of Health Preservation* said that "from Summer Solstice to Autumnal Equinox, people should avoid eating greasy cakes and pastries, which are very similar to wine, melons and fruits, and many diseases in summer are caused by them", indicating that people should not eat greasy and sweet food that is hard to digest in summer; otherwise it will lead to diseases. Food is perishable in summer, so we should pay attention to food hygiene to prevent the occurrence of intestinal infectious diseases. There is a record in *The Analects of Confucius* that "do not eat it when the color of the food has changed. Do not eat it when the smell of the food has changed. Do not eat it if the food is improperly cooked. Do not eat it if the food is not in time. Do not eat it if the meat is not properly cut". There is also a record in *Synopsis of Golden Chamber* that "dirty rice, decomposed meat and smelly fish can all hurt the body if taken".

How do people take medications for health preservation in summer?

People easily suffer from heatstroke, diarrhea and other diseases in summer. TCM also advocates using medication to prevent diseases. For instance, drinking mung bean soup and Huangqi (Astragali Radix) water can clear summer heat and replenish qi, promote production of fluid and quench thirst. *Key Points of Syndrome and Treatment* also advocates taking Heye (Nelumbinis Folium) porridge regularly, which has the effect of preventing heatstroke. From the Grain Full to the Lesser Heat, many heat diseases may occur, which can be prevented by oral administration of water-decocted Maidong (Ophiopogonis Radix), Jinyinhua (Lonicerae Japonicae Flos), Lianqiao (Forsythiae Fructus), Wuweizi (Schisandrae Chinensis Fructus), Dangshen (Codonopsis Radix), Fuling (Poria) and Gancao (Glycyrrhizae Radix et Rhizoma); from the Greater Heat to the White Dew, people are easy to suffer from dampness diseases, which can be prevented by oral administration of water-decocted Biandou (Lablab Semen Album), Yiyiren (Coicis Semen), Guanghuoxiang (Pogostemonis Herba) and Shengdihuang (Rehmanniae Radix). In addition, for some chronic diseases that often occur or worsen in winter, such as emphysema, asthma and diarrhea, TCM advocates "treating winter diseases in summer", which can play an ideal role in preventing and treating diseases.

ⅠⅠⅠ Health preservation in autumn

What are the climate characteristics of autumn?

Huangdi Neijing said: "The three months of autumn are the period in which the shapes of everything are formed gloriously and peacefully. The heaven qi becomes swift, while the earth qi becomes clear. In autumn, it is desirable to sleep early and get up early at the crowing of a rooster. It is desirable to maintain a peaceful will in autumn in order to slow down the killing effects of the autumn. It is desirable to constrict energy of spirits in order to restrict the killing effects of the autumn. It is also desirable to refrain from moving into the outside world so that the energy of the lungs remains clean and clear. This is the good style to maintain in response to the autumn in order to rejuvenate and harvest. To live a lifestyle contrary to the autumn will cause harm to the lungs and one will suffer diarrhea with undigested foods in winter that follows, because there is a shortage of energy to store away in winter."

The three months of autumn begin at the Beginning of Autumn and end at the Beginning of Winter. Autumn is the season of harvest when everything is mature and fruitful. When it comes to autumn, the yang between heaven and earth recedes day by day, the yin and cold gradually grow, and the climate gradually turns cool. The climate changes greatly in the morning and night, and freezing air often attacks. Yang qi gradually converges, and yin qi gradually grows. The scenery gradually develops into a state of depression, and yang qi of the human body also converges.

How do people cultivate the spirit in autumn?

In autumn, the air is crisp, and the climate is getting colder. The autumn wind is strong, and the earth qi is clear. All living beings are decaying, which makes people feel sad and worried. The corresponding viscera of autumn are the lungs, and sorrow and worries are the most likely to hurt the lungs. Therefore, to cultivate the spirit, people should be quiet and calm in the heart, peaceful in mind, and comfortable in the mood. People should not be sad and worried. They can climb high mountains to enjoy the sight of chrysanthemums and watch red leaves, so as to please the mental state.

How do people recuperate daily life in autumn?

In autumn, people should "go to bed early and get up early, which is similar to the timetable of chickens". Going to bed early is to adapt to the convergence of yin essence, and getting up early is to adapt to the relaxation of yang. Autumn climate is characterized by dryness, low humidity in the air and strong wind, which often makes people's skin dry. We should keep a certain humidity in the room, and pay attention to replenishing water in the body to avoid impairment of fluid by sweating. The temperature is changeable in autumn, and the temperatures in the morning and evening differ largely, so people should pay attention to increasing or decreasing clothes at any time. Autumn is also a good time to exercise. Exercise in autumn should be focused on static work, such as internal qigong and Yishougong. According to the characteristics that autumn dryness can easily hurt the lungs, methods such as "knocking the teeth", "laying the tongue against palate", "swallowing the fluid", and "guhe (taking deep breath)" can be adopted to preserve health. The dynamic exercise can also be properly adopted, such as Wuqinxi, Baduanjin and Taijiquan. In addition, in autumn, people can gradually do some cold-resistant exercises, such as cold baths.

How do people recuperate by diet in autumn?

The guiding ideology of dietetic conditioning is to prevent dryness and protect yin, nourish kidney and moisten lung, and take "less pungent and more acid" as the principle. *Synopsis of Golden Chamber* pointed out that "people should not eat food that corresponds to the lungs in autumn", because the lung qi is too strong in autumn and should not be further supplemented. *Key to Diet* said that "the qi in autumn is dry, people should eat sesame to moisten the dryness". Therefore, people should eat less pungent and dry products such as pepper, onion, scallion and garlic, and eat more soft and moistening things such as sesame, glutinous rice, honey, sugar cane, spinach and dairy products. The elderly can also eat porridge in the morning to benefit stomach and promote production of fluid. *Introduction to Medicine* recorded that "eating porridge in the morning can get rid of the stale and bring forth thefresh, benefit diaphragm and nourish stomach, and generate body fluid, which makes people feel refreshed for a day, showing great replenishing effect". Baihe (Lilii Bulbus) Lianzi (Nelumbinis Semen) porridge, Yin'er (Tremella fuciformis) sugar porridge,

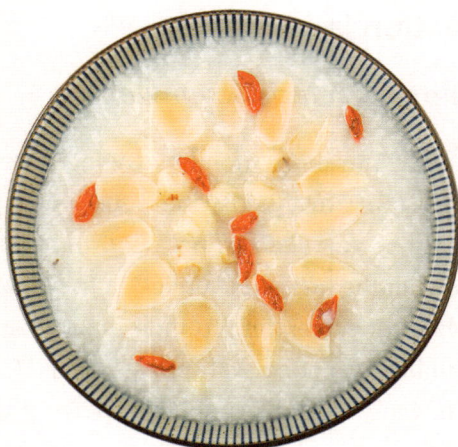

Baihe Lianzi porridge

jujube and glutinous rice porridge, fresh Dihuang (Rehmanniae Radix) juice porridge, black sesame porridge, etc. in TCM are all good products in autumn that benefit yin and nourish stomach and can be taken multiple times and for a long time.

How do people take medications for health preservation in autumn?

According to the climate characteristics in autumn, people can usually take Renshen (Ginseng Radix et Rhizoma), Shashen (Glehniae Radix), Maidong (Ophiopogonis Radix), Baihe (Lilii Bulbus), Xingren (Armeniacae Semen Amarum), Chuanbeimu (Fritillariae Cirrhosae Bulbus), Pangdahai (Sterculiae Lychnophorae Semen) and other traditional Chinese medicinals with effects of benefiting qi and nourishing yin, and ventilating lung qi to dissipate phlegm. Dryness disease is easy to occur from the Autumnal Equinox to the Beginning of Winter, which can be prevented by oral administration of Shengdihuang (Rehmanniae Radix), Baihe (Lilii Bulbus), Dangshen (Codonopsis Radix), Fengmi (Mel), Maidong (Ophiopogonis Radix) and Gancao (Glycyrrhizae Radix et Rhizoma).

IV Health preservation in winter

What are the climate characteristics of winter?

Huangdi Neijing said: "The three months of winter are the period in which everything is closed and stored away. In winter, the water freezes and the earth cracks. Yang energy should be guarded and not be disturbed. It is desirable to sleep early and get up late, to wait the arrival of sunlight. One should tightly guard one's emotions as if hiding them or pretending to hide them, not unlike someone with private intentions, not unlike someone with private gains. One should avoid cold and stay close to warm. One should refrain from perspiring, which will deprive the body of its yang energy. This is the good style to maintain in response to winter in order to rejuvenate and put things in storage. To live a lifestyle contrary to the winter causes harm to the kidneys, and one will suffer from wei (atrophy) with weak and cold limbs in the spring that follows, because there is a shortage of energy to generate in spring due to poor storage in the preceding winter."

The three months of winter start at the Beginning of Winter and end at the Beginning of Spring. Winter is the season when everything is preserved and stored, with abundant yin and latent yang, withered plants, dormant insects, frozen earth, cold climate, and accident cold-air outbreak. Therefore, yang qi of the human body is hidden inside.

How do people cultivate the spirit in winter?

When winter comes, everything is withering. The corresponding viscus of winter is the kidney. Spirit cultivation in winter should focus on being quiet and reserved. The latent yang qi should not be disturbed. People should especially pay attention to avoiding cold and keeping warm, so as to preserve yang qi. And enjoying the snow scenery can contribute to people's peace of mind or inner tranquility.

How do people recuperate daily life in winter?

The weather is freezing in winter, so the principle of health preservation should be to avoid cold and keep warm, and to preserve yang and protect yin. In terms of daily life, it is necessary to "go to bed early and get up late till the sun shines", "avoid cold as well as wind in winter" (*Primary Mirror of Rectifying Deficiency*), so the indoor temperature should be kept warm; in terms of clothing, we should take warmth, comfort and good circulation of qi and blood as the principle. In addition, during the closure and storage of winter, it is rather important to consolidate the mind, preserve the essence and nourish the mind. Therefore, TCM pays special attention to the control of sexual intercourse in winter. *Zunsheng Bajian* pointed out that "the three months in winter are a good chance to cultivate viscera, and people's spirit should also be reserved"; the ancients even advocated that sexual intercourse should be "once in spring, twice in summer, once in autumn and none in winter", which fully explains the importance of controlling sexual intercourse and protecting yin essence in response to the features of winter. In winter, people should also overcome the difficulties of cold climate and actively participate in fitness exercises.

How do people recuperate by diet in winter?

The guiding ideology of health preservation in winter is "protecting yin and nurturing yang". The principle of diet is "less salty". *Key to Diet* said that "winter is cold, so it is advisable to eat millet to treat cold with heat", which advocates eating hot food. However, it should be noticed that hot and dry food should be eaten in moderation, so as to avoid internal yang depression transforming into heat. Of course, raw and cold food should also be avoided. People are recommended to eat more mutton, turtle, lotus root, agaric, sesame and other food. The flavor of food can be properly stronger, and carrots, spinach, bean sprout and other fresh vegetables can be eaten more. In winter, the amount of activity is small, and the metabolism of the human body slows down. Therefore, people cannot eat too much. After meal, people can rub the abdomen to help with food transformation.

How do people take medications for health preservation in winter?

Winter governs closure and storage. "Winter stores the essence". Winter is a good time to supplement. However, choosing food supplements or drug supplements should be carried out under the guidance of doctors according to people's own conditions, and they should not be blindly conducted. Under normal circumstances, for those with deficiency of yang, mutton and chicken are the main food supplements, and Renshen (Ginseng Radix et Rhizoma), Lurong (Cervi Cornu Pantotrichum), Jingui Shenqi Pills and other prescriptions can also be used for drug supplements; for those with deficiency of yin and blood, duck meat, goose meat, pork liver, agaric, etc. can be used for food supplements, and Ejiao (Asini Corii Colla), Danggui (Angelicae Sinensis Radix), Gouqizi (Lycii Fructus) and Liuwei Dihuang Pills can be used for drug supplements. In addition, those who are physically weak should not be strongly or even vigorously supplemented, but should be replenished step by step. For those who are physically healthy, it is best to use food supplements, and it is better to take drug supplements to tonify the body mildly in winter; for those with weak constitutions, it is advised for them to pay equal attention to food supplements and drug supplements, and conduct supplement under the guidance of doctors.

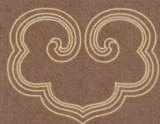

Chapter 4

Cultivating the Spirit

Section 1
Unity of the Body and Spirit

What is the body?What is the spirit?

TCM holds that the human body is composed of "body" and "spirit". The so-called "body" refers to the whole body structure of a person, including organizational structures such as internal viscera, meridians and collaterals, limbs and bones, and basic nutrients such as qi, blood, fluid and essence, which are the material basis. The so-called "spirit" can be divided into a broad sense and a narrow sense. In the broad sense, the spirit refers to the whole life activity phenomenon, including language, sight, body movement, posture and the image of the whole human body; while in the narrow sense, the spirit refers to the spirit dominated by the heart in TCM, including human spirit, consciousness, characteristics, emotion and other activities, which are functions.

What is the unity of the body and spirit?

Zhang Jingyue pointed out in the *Classified Canon*: "The body is the quality of the spirit, and the spirit is the application of the body; the spirit cannot live without the body, and vice versa." He also said: "People are born with the qi of yin and yang in the heaven and earth, and they are formed by flesh and blood. The qi flow in the body to become the spirit. The body and spirit thus form a whole." "Unity of the body and spirit" is the life view of TCM, which is also called "harmony of body and spirit" or "the accordance of the body and spirit". That is, the integration of the body and spirit. The spirit of TCM not only dominates people's spiritual activities, but also dominates people's material metabolism and energy metabolism. Although spirit is transformed from essence and qi, it in turn dominates essence and qi activities, which shows that the body and spirit depend on each other, influence each other and are inseparable.

How to cultivate the body with the spirit?

Spirit plays a dominant and regulating role in the overall function. TCM health preservation experts think that regulating spirit is the first priority, and the functional state of spirit determines the success or failure of health preservation. *Basic Questions–Linglan Midian Lun* recorded: "The heart is the monarch organ where the spirit comes out." *Basic Questions–Tiaojing Lun* said: "The heart storage the spirit." TCM believes that the spirit is the master of human activities, the generation of spirit can be attributed to five zang viscera, but it is generally governed by the heart. Therefore, spirit cultivation is heart cultivation. If the heart is properly nurtured, then "if the monarch is wise, its subordinates will be stable and normal. If people use this principle for health preservation, they can live a long life without danger. If they use it to govern the world, they will make the country prosperous". If the heart is under malnutrition, then "if the monarch is unwise, then all the twelve viscera, including itself, will be in danger. And the way for each viscera to play its normal role will be blocked, and the body will be seriously damaged. In this case, talking about health preservation will only lead to disasters. Similarly, if the monarch governs the world with ignorance, the regime will be in danger". Ji Kang, a health preserver in the Three Kingdoms Period, also put forward the health preservation thought of "cultivating the nature to protect the spirit, and keeping peace in the mind to protect the body". To sum up, preserving the heart and spirit is the priority of health preservation.

How can we achieve the coexistence of the body and spirit?

Nourishing both the body and spirit is the greatest method of health preservation recommended by TCM. *Huangdi Neijing* clearly put forward the viewpoint of "harmony of body and spirit". For example, *Basic Questions–Shanggu Tianzhen Lun* said: "In this way, the harmony of body and spirit can be achieved, and people can live to an expected longevity and die after a hundred years old." In addition, it put forward the method of "timely avoiding pathogens" to tonify the body externally, and "being indifferent to fame or gain, keepiing inside the essence and spirit" to nourish the genuine qi to supplement the spirit internally. *Basic Questions–Siqi Tiaoshen Dalun* further recorded the exercise method of nourishing both the body and spirit in accordance with the different climates of spring, summer, autumn and winter. For example, in the three months of spring, for body cultivation, "people should go to bed at night and get up early, walk casually in yard, lovsen their hair, untie their clothes, and relax their bodies", so as to nourish the spirit and achieve "keeping everything alive".

TCM health preservation has a long history, and there are various specific health preservation methods. However, it can be summed up as "body cultivation" and "spirit cultivation". That is, the so-called "preserving the spirit to complete the body" and "preserving the body to complete the spirit". Whether it is "body completion" or "spirit completion", it is achieved through nourishing both the body and spirit, so as to make the spirit prosper and protect the body, thus achieving longevity.

Section 2
Emotional Health Preservation

What is the impact of seven excessive emotions on the human body?

Basic Questions–Tianyuanji Dalun said: "The five zang viscera develop five qi as joy, anger, sorrow, worry, and fear." Emotions in TCM refer to seven emotions of joy, anger, worry, thought, sorrow, fright and fear. Emotions are generated by the qi of the five zang viscera. Therefore, TCM believes that emotional activities are closely related to viscera; excessive emotional activities can also cause diseases in viscera, which are mainly manifested as follows: first, abnormal qi movement. For example, *Basic Questions–Jutong Lun* holds that "all diseases are caused by the changes of qi. Anger leads to qi ascending, joy leads to qi loose, sorrow leads to qi elimination, fear leads to qi sinking, cold leads to qi contraction, heat leads to qi dispersion, fright leads to qi turbulence, overexertion leads to qi consumption, and thought leads to qi knotting". Second, imbalance of yin and yang. *Basic Questions–Shuwuguo Lun* said: "Excessive anger hurts yin, and excessive joy hurts yang. The reversed qi goes upward and fills in the meridians. The spirit also floats outward and leaves the body." That is to say, excessive anger damages the yin of the human body, while excessive joy consumes yang qi. *Miraculous Pivot–Baibing Shisheng* said: "If people lose control of their emotions, the viscera will be hurt, which indicates that the disease originates in yin." It believes that if there is no moderation of emotions, the five zang viscera will be hurt. The five zang viscera pertain to yin, so the disease is believed to start from yin if the five zang viscera are hurt. Third, loss of essence and blood. *Introduction to Medicine* recorded that "overwhelming joy will disturb the heart and impair the heart's function of governing blood", which means that excessive joy will damage heart qi. TCM believes that one of the functions of heart is that heart governs blood, and the heart with the impairment of heart qi can't govern blood, resulting in the probable occurrence of blood deficiency, blood stasis and other blood syndromes. Fourth, direct visceral damage. *Basic Questions–Yinyang Yingxiang Dalun* said: "Anger impairs the liver, joy impairs the heart, thought impairs the spleen, worry impairs Rage lung, and fear impairs the kidney." It vividly illustrated the influence of different excessive emotions on the corresponding viscera. Fifth, a series of symptoms. Chao Yuanfang's *General Treatise on Causes and Manifestations of All*

Diseases in the Sui Dynasty said: "Anger can make qi go upward and impair heart qi, leading to shortness of breath and feeling of impending death. Grievance can result in qi accumulation below the heart. People thus don't feel like eating. Worry can inhibit the sudden movement of qi, and people can't lie peacefully at night. Joy makes people unable to run and stand forlong. Anxiety makes people lose the ability to distinguish people, toss things everywhere, and can't get anywhere. If people hear urgent news, they will feel stiffness in the four limbs and cannot lift them up." It means that people will feel dry heat and shortness of breath when angry. Grievance is easy to accumulate in the stomach, and people tend to fail to eat food. Worry can lead to insomnia, and so on.

How do people apply emotional health preservation appropriately?

In regard of emotional health preservation, it is necessary to achieve "harmonizing emotions and adjusting rigidity and softness". *Miraculous Pivot– Benshen* said: "A wise person's health-preserving method must conform to the changes of climates of four seasons, harmonize emotions and adjust daily life, control yin and yang and adjust rigidity and softness. Only in this way can people not be invaded by exopathogens, and achieve longevity." There is a saying in *Qian Gongliang Ceyu*: "If people don't get angry when they are encountered with angry things, and don't get ecstatic when faced with happy things, in this way, a good mind can be cultivated." In addition, the famous viewpoint of "Eight Bases and Three Good Fortune" is recorded in *Home-Letters from Zeng Guofan*. The "Eight Bases" refer to "reading ancient books should take exegesis as the base, writing poems and compositions should take tones as the base, providing for the elderly should take their favors as the base, health preservation should take less anger as the base, conducting ourselves in society should be based on not talking nonsense, managing a family should be based on not getting up late, being an official should be based on not being greedy for money, and marching is based on not disturbing civilians", among which "health preservation should take less anger as the base" is also about harmonizing and adjusting emotions. "Three virtues for auspiciousness" refers to filial piety, diligence, and forgiveness. It is believed that being filial to parents, being diligent and frugal, and treating others with kindness and generosity are virtuous behaviors that can bring blessings to the family and must be followed.

Section 3
Mind Cultivation

Why is it so important to cultivate people's mind?

Ancient Chinese health preservation doctors always paid attention to the cultivation of mind, and thought that people live between heaven and earth, and their mentality plays a vital role in the rise and fall, and gain and loss of the whole body. Therefore, ancient health preservation experts put special emphasis on cultivating the mind and improving morality. The ancients believed that "health preservation first give priority to mind cultivation", which refers to self-cultivation. Confucianism, Buddhism and Taoism also attach great importance to self-cultivation, mind-body co-cultivation, nature-life co-cultivation. Confucianism believes that it is very important to nurture, cultivate, and educate the mind in the process of cultivating the body, managing the family, governing the country and ruling the world. *The Great Learning* said: "Knowledge can be acquired only after understanding and studying everything; after acquiring knowledge, the mind can be sincere; only when the mind is sincere can the mind be correct; only when the mind is correct can people cultivate the body and mind; only after the cultivation of the body and mind can people manage the family and house well; only by managing families and houses can people govern the country well; only when the country is well governed can the world be peaceful."

How do people cultivate the mind?

In the cultivation of mind, the most important thing is to be pure in heart and reduce desires. *Huangdi Neijing* holds that "being indifferent to fame or gain, the genuine qi will follow the direction, and the essence and spirit are kept inside. Where can the disease come from? The mind is leisurely with few desires, stable with no fear, and the body is tired but not worn out". Mencius also put forward a similar view, holding that "for mind cultivation, there is nothing better than having few desires". That is to say, if people want to keep a peaceful mind and not to be greedy for delusions, they can keep their spirit healthy and prosperous, and thus prevent diseases. In order to achieve less selfishness and few desires, ancient sages also advocated "suppressing eyes and silencing ears", because eyes and ears are the main approaches for human body to contact with external stimuli. Once eyes are clear and ears are quiet, the spirit and qi will be kept inside and the heart will not be bothered. If eyes are flashed and ears are disturbed, the spirit and qi will be exhausted and the heart will be worried. *A Supplement to Recipes Worth A Thousand Gold* pointed out that "the key to health preservation lies in not listening to things that should not be heard, not saying things that should not be said, not doing things that should not be done, and not thinking about things that should not be considered, all of which are conducive to health preservation".

The ancients also believed that nature cultivation can prolong life, and only by paying attention to morality cultivation in health preservation can we enter the domain of benevolence and longevity. Confucius clearly pointed out in *The Doctrine of the Mean* that "to correct oneself, one must strengthen the moral quality. And to strengthen moral quality, benevolence must be regarded as the priority. Only when people have noble moral quality can they live a long life". There is saying in *The Great Learning* that "wealth can decorate the house, while morality can decorate the body and mind". *The Analects of Confucius* said: "Wise people are happy, and benevolent people live long." *Zunsheng Bajian* by Gao Lian in the Ming Dynasty said: "Those who are good at health preservation do it on the inside; those who are not good at health preservation do it on the outside. Being greedy for the outside happiness will weaken the inside. The so-called inside cultivation will calm the five zang viscera, keep sanjiao in place, instruct proper diet, and eliminate mundane matters, leading to longevity." It provides us with some instructions of practical implementation. Gong Tingxian, a doctor in the Ming Dynasty, said in his book *Prolonging Life and Preserving the Origin*: "Accumulating good deeds and always preserving hidden virtue can prolong life." All the above were considered by the ancients to achieve the purpose of prolonging life.

How does qigong guide the cultivation of the mind?

There is a special form of mind cultivation—qigong. The word qigong has existed since ancient times. In *Records of Jingming Religion* written by Xu Xun in the Jin Dynasty, there was a name of "qigong chanwei". In the ancient books before the Jin Dynasty, Taoism called it "tuna" and "liandan". Confucianism called it "zhengxin" and "xiushen". Buddhism called it "canchan", "zhiguan", "dazuo" and "ruding", and doctors called it "daoyin" and "shesheng". Even some martial arts such as Taijiquan belong to the scope of qigong as long as they are based on internal strength. Qigong mainly integrates the body and mind by adjusting posture, exercising breathing, relaxing the body and mind, controlling consciousness, exercising the body rhythmically, etc., so as to achieve the predetermined exercise purpose. It means that through introverted application of consciousness, self-consciousness activities and life activities are combined, which enhances the life activities of the body and inspires the inner potential of the human body, thus playing the role of cultivating the mood, developing wisdom, preventing and treating diseases and prolonging life. It includes three aspects: body adjustment (posture adjustment), respiration adjustment (breathing adjustment) and heart adjustment (mind stability).

What are the ten pleasures?

Pleasant feelings and smooth spirits require rich and colorful life arrangements, and cultivation of elegant hobbies and noble sentiments, so as to maintain a "persistent happy" state of mind. Xu Chunfu said in *The Medical Encyclopedia in Ancient and Modern Times:* "It is in people's nature to be addicted to things. There are people who like painting and calligraphy, piano and chess, games, treasures, medicines, birds and horses, and antiquities...which make them enjoy themselves." Ten pleasures were recorded in *The New Book of Providing for the Aged*: reading to understand the truths, learning calligraphy, clearing mind and sitting quietly, chatting with good friends, sipping, watering flowers and planting bamboo, listening to the *guqin* (a plucked seven-string Chinese musical instrument) and playing with cranes, burning incense and boiling tea, boating and enjoying the views of mountains, and being devoted to playing chess. Gao Tongxuan, a painter in the Qing Dynasty, also had "ten pleasures": the joy of ploughing and weeding, brooming, teaching children, being content, peaceful living, free talking, rambling, bathing, leisurely lying, and exposing the back to the sun.

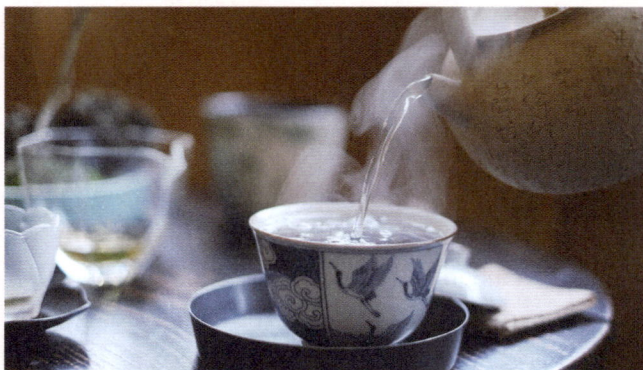

Drinking tea

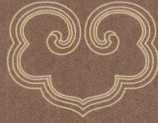

Chapter 5

Dietetic Health Preservation

Section 1
Overview of Dietetic Health Preservation

What is dietetic health preservation?

Dietetic health preservation, also known as "dietary nutrition", is a method of maintaining health, prolonging life, and assisting in the prevention and treatment of diseases using the properties of food, guided by the basic TCM principles. It involves studying the characteristics of different foods and utilizing them to support health, as well as to complement medical treatments and prevent disease recurrence.

What are the contents of dietetic health preservation?

Dietetic health preservation, based on historical literature and clinical practice, mainly includes three aspects: maintaining health, preventing and treating diseases, and post-treatment prevention of recurrence. It also involves two methods: dietary moderation and dietary do's and don'ts.

Reasonable diet, also known as "dietary nutrition" or "dietary supplementation", refers to the use of diet to nourish the body, maintain or enhance health. The concept of "nutrition therapy" is early recorded in the ancient medical text *Basic Questions–Wuchangzheng Dalun,* which states, "Grains, meat, fruits, and vegetables, are all used for dietary nutrition."

Using diet to prevent and treat diseases is known as "dietary therapy" or "dietary treatment", which refers to the use of diet to treat or complement medical treatment for diseases. In the book *Essential Recipes for Emergent Use Worth A Thousand Gold–Dietary Therapy*, Sun Simiao wrote: "Food can expel pathogenic factors, harmonize the organs, please the spirit, and invigorate the will, thereby nourishing the blood and qi." This reflects the dual role of dietary therapy in expelling pathogenic factors and supporting the body's vitality. Subsequently, specialized works on dietary therapy, such as *Materia Medica for Dietetic Therapy*, were published.

Dietary adjustment for post-treatment recovery and prevention of recurrence refers to the use of dietary moderation and dietary do's and don'ts, tailored to the individual's condition, to promote quick recovery and prevent disease recurrence. In *Basic Questions–Re Lun*, it is stated, "When the disease is still not fully resolved, eating meat will cause relapse; excessive eating will lead to lingering illness." This passage specifically explains the dietary considerations during the recovery phase of febrile diseases.

Why did ancient doctors pay equal attention to food and medicines?

Shennong's Classic of Materia Medica, the first pharmaceutical monograph in China, contains 365 kinds of TCM medicinals, many of which are both medicines and food. There are categories of "dietetician", "general medicine" and "royal surgeon" recorded in *Rites of Zhou–Tianguan*, and the "dieteticians" are the doctors who are especially in charge of dietetic health preservation and food hygiene. *Basic Questions–Wuchangzheng Dalun* pointed out that after the disease was relieved, "the patient should be supplemented by the grain, meat, fruits and vegetables" to facilitate the recovery after the disease. *Basic Questions–Zangqi Fashi Lun* said that "five grains are used for nourishment, five fruits facilitate the nourishment, five livestock are used for tonification, and five vegetables are used for supplement. If they are taken in accordance with their qi and flavors, the essence and qi can be supplemented", which shows that the ancients advocated the combination of food and medicines in the treatment process. Zhang Zhongjing, a doctor in the Eastern Han Dynasty, used many foods to treat diseases. For example, Zhufu Decoction and Danggui Shengjiang Mutton Decoction recorded in *Treatise on Cold Damage* and *Synopsis of Golden Chamber* are typical special prescriptions for dietetic therapy. In the Tang Dynasty, *Essential Recipes for Emergent Use Worth A Thousand Gold* and *A Supplement to Recipes Worth A Thousand Gold* compiled by Sun Simiao respectively set up a special volume on "Dietetic Therapy" and a special section on "Dietary Therapy for the Elderly", put forward that "when treating a disease, a doctor must first treat it with food according to the cause of the disease and the viscera invaded, and then treat it with medicines if the dietetic therapy fails to heal", and quoted Bian Que's saying that "the essence of living is diet, and the only key to relieve emergency is medicines. People who don't know the compatibility and incompatibility of diet cannot preserve their health...When there is a disease, it should be treated with food first, and then medicine if dietetic therapy does not work".

What are the monographs of ancient dietetic therapy?

Materia Medica for Dietetic Therapy, written by Meng Shen in the Tang Dynasty, is the first monograph on dietetic therapy in China, which is a great collection of dietetic therapy before the Tang Dynasty. Another monograph on dietetic therapy in the Tang Dynasty is Zan Yin's *Reflections on Dietotherapy,* which collected about more than 200 dietetic therapy prescriptions, including soup, fried food, porridge, wonton, cake, tea, wine, etc. It paid special attention to porridge therapy, recording 57 prescriptions of medicinal porridge, which laid the foundation of medicinal porridge therapy for later generations. Since then, there have been monographs on dietetic health preservation, such as *Key to Diet, The New Book of Providing for the Aged, Identification of Materia Medica, Recipe at Home* and *Identification Record of Diet,* which show that people have always valued dietetic health preservation. *The New Book of Providing for the Aged* in the Yuan Dynasty said: "If people know the nature of their food and use them appropriately, it will be twice better than taking medicines." It can be seen that dietetic health preservation is an important part of the treasure house of TCM, which has made contributions to the prevention and treatment of diseases, health care, cooking and nutrition of the Chinese nation, and is one of the important methods of health preservation.

What is the harm of improper dietetic health preservation?

There has always been a saying that "medicinal supplement is no better than dietetic supplement", but the dietetic supplement is not available to everyone, nor can it be applied to every disease. In *Synopsis of Golden Chamber,* the impact of improper diet on the body was especially emphasized, saying, "Diet is for the nourishment of the body. If the diet is taken improperly, it can do harm to the body... the harm will become the disease, thus leading to danger."

Section 2
Diet Based on Syndrome Differentiation

How do people give attention to both spleen and stomach function when applying dietetic health preservation?

When the spleen and stomach function is vigorous, the patients can be supplemented with dietetic nutrition in accordance with the needs of recovery from the disease. For example, for patients with weak constitutions and severe anemia, medicinals with an affinity with flesh and blood can be selected for supplement, and high-protein food and animal livers can be chosen to replenish the blood. If the spleen and stomach function of the patient is weak, with decreased appetite, abdominal distention, loose stool and thick and greasy tongue coating, "treating deficiency syndrome with tonifying methods" should not be emphasized. Eating too much will add to the burden on the spleen and stomach. If the patient is "too weak to be tonified", a light diet should be selected to regulate the spleen and stomach first. After the recovery of the spleen and stomach function, the dietetic supplement can be applied.

How do people apply dietetic health preservation in accordance with individuality?

Synopsis of Golden Chamber said that "people with internal heat should not eat mutton". "Pregnant women should not eat rabbit meat...it will result in muteness of her baby". Although these statements need further study, it shows that dietetic health preservation must vary from person to person. For example, cock, pig's head meat, etc., are tonic for ordinary people, but are not suitable for those who suffer from intermittent headaches and headaches with the syndrome of upward disturbance of liver yang. Taking them can induce chronic diseases; there are also some people with special qualities, with allergies to seafood, fish, shrimp and crab, which can cause allergic reactions and induce urticaria, asthma and other diseases.

How do people apply dietetic health preservation in accordance with local conditions?

Huangdi Neijing pointed out that the eastern region is a land of fish and salt.

People there "eat fish and are addicted to salt", "fish cause internal heat, and salt hurts blood", and the common disease there is "swollen sore" (*Basic Questions–Yifa Fangyi Lun*), which shows that dietetic health preservation must be adapted to local conditions. For example, to supplement in winter, food with strong warm and supplementary nature, such as mutton and venison, is suitable for the freezing weather; while the climate in the south is mild, food with sweet, warm and supplementary nature, such as pork, chicken, duck and fish, can be chosen. People who work on water for a long time or live by the sea are often invaded by dampness exopathogen, so dietetic health preservation must be accompanied by traditional Chinese medicinals with the effect of invigorating spleen to eliminate dampness. People who work at high altitudes for a long time or live in mountainous areas are often invaded by dryness exopathogen, so dietetic health preservation must be accompanied by traditional Chinese medicinals with clear, cold, dispersing and moistening nature, such as tremella, rock sugar, pear, soft-shelled turtle and tortoise.

How do people apply dietetic health preservation in accordance with seasonal conditions?

The ancients paid great attention to applying dietetic health preservation in accordance with seasonal conditions. *Qianjin Shizhi–Preface* said: "From the Summer Solstice to the Autumnal Equinox, people must be careful of fatty, cake-like and greasy food." It also said: "During the 72 days of spring, people should eat less sour food and more sweet food to nourish spleen qi; during the 72 days of summer, people should eat less bitter food and more pungent food to nourish lung qi; during the 72 days of autumn, people should eat less pungent food and more sour food to nourish liver qi; during the 72 days of winter, people should eat less salty food and more bitter food to nourish heart qi; in the last month of each season, eat sweet food and more salty food to cultivate to nourish kidney qi." It can be seen that dietetic health preservation should be adjusted according to the seasonal changes in the four seasons. Another example is that in summer, the elderly with weak constitutions can't stand the heat because of their reduced adaptability. In addition to paying attention to preventing sunstroke, they are advised to eat some nourishment products with cold nature, such as mung bean porridge and Heye (Nelumbinis Folium) porridge, which can not only relieve summer heat, but also promote production of fluid and quench thirst. In the cold winter, people's yang qi is likely to get hurt. The yang qi of the elderly is deficient, so they are suggested to eat some nourishment products with warm and tonic nature to warm yang to dispel cold, such as mutton porridge and Roucongrong (Cistanches Herba) porridge.

How do people formulate a diet according to syndrome differentiation?

Due to different physical conditions, living habits and symptoms, the weak conditions and the nature of the disease are also different. Therefore, for dietetic health preservation, people must identify the cold and heat, deficiency and excess of the disease, the loss of qi, blood, yin and yang of zang and fu viscera, and select dietetic health preservation products with the effects of invigorating qi, blood, yin, yang, heart, liver, spleen, lung and kidney. For people with yin deficiency, food should be light and tonic, such as Baihe (Lilii Bulbus), Guijia (Testudinis Carapax et Plastrum), sea cucumber and tremella; for people with yang deficiency, food with warm and tonic nature such as mutton and venison can be used.

The purpose of dietetic health preservation is to achieve a "relative equilibrium of yin and yang", and to adjust the yin, yang, qi and blood of the zang and fu viscera of the body to achieve balance. Therefore, the treatment is not simply replenishing qi for qi deficiency, enriching blood for blood deficiency, nourishing yin for yin deficiency, or strengthening yang for yang deficiency. Because replenishing qi too much can lead to stagnation of qi and abnormal ascending and descending activity; nourishing yin too much can restrain yang qi, and aggravate yin cold. Therefore, when tonifying qi, blood should be replenished as well, and when replenishing blood, qi should be tonified as well. Nourishing yin needs to be accompanied by warming yang, and yin fluid needs to be protected. In this way, the balance of yin and yang, and qi and blood can be achieved.

Medicated diet is a combination of medicine and food, which presents a synergistic effect. Food, like medicine, is born with the qi of yin and yang in heaven and earth. Both of them have nature, flavor, ascending and descending, and meridian tropism, which are also called medicinal properties and food properties. Because of the difference in medicinal properties and food properties, their functions are different. Before applying diet, the medicinals and food should be correctly selected based on syndrome differentiation according to the symptoms and constitutions of the eaters, combined with the different geographical environments, living habits and seasons. By "combining medicinals based on prescriptions, formulating prescriptions based on principles, setting principles based on theories and establishing theories based on evidence", the expected purpose can be achieved. Medicated diet is shaped like food and has the same nature as medicines. Medicated diet is a kind of substance which takes food as the carrier and is processed and produced by cooking methods similar to food, so that medicines and food can play a certain role together. It is different from both general food and general medicines. Like food, it has sensory properties such as color, aroma and flavor, and like medicines, it has the characteristics of being safe, non-toxic and effective. The two are combined and cooperate with each other to achieve the purpose of "the medicine taking advantage of food and food helping the medicine with supplement".

How do people apply medicated diet?

Application principles for middle-aged people: middle age is a turning point from prosperity to decline. The functions of viscera are gradually declining. Especially the nerves are gradually deficient, adding to the great pressure of life and work, which leads to the consumption of yin and blood and the decline of visceral functions, presenting dizziness, palpitation, fatigue, memory decline, sexual dysfunction, and even premature aging. Health care and physical fitness in this period are particularly important. For menopausal women, a medicated diet with effects of dispersing liver and regulating qi can be used, and it has the functions of relieving menopausal symptoms, and strengthening and beautifying skin after long-term application.

Application principle for the elderly: the visceral functions of the elderly have declined, and there are often a series of deficiency syndromes such as deficiency of qi and blood, deficiency of kidney essence, deficiency of spleen and fluid, qi deficiency and phlegm coagulation, and qi deficiency and phlegm stasis, presenting dizziness, palpitation, shortness of breath, fatigue, insomnia, dreaminess, loss of appetite, forgetfulness, tinnitus, sexual hypofunction, constipation, etc. Medicinals with the effects of replenishing essence and marrow, invigorating qi and blood, strengthening waist and kidney, invigorating qi and promoting blood circulation should be selected.

Section 3
Harmonizing Five Flavors

What are the characteristics of food in terms of nature and taste?

The characteristics of food mainly refer to its temperature, which can be categorized as cold, hot, warm, and cool, and the taste mainly refers to its flavor, which can be categorized as sour, bitter, sweet, spicy, and salty.

How can we utilize the nature of food for dietetic health preservation?

The hot and cold natures of medicinal substances are two opposing attributes. The essence of dietetic health preservation is to use the nature of food to correct the imbalances in the body. The general principle of TCM is "treating coldness with warmth and treating warmth with coldness". The same principle applies to dietary adjustment, where individuals with a hot constitution or those suffering from heat-related conditions should consume cool/cold foods rather than hot foods, while individuals with a cold constitution or those suffering from cold-related conditions should consume hot foods rather than cold foods.

Common hot foods include chili peppers, Sichuan peppercorns, ginger, garlic, onions, alcohol, longan fruit, mutton, and rooster meat, while common cold foods include mung beans, white radish, tofu, water chestnuts, crabs, soft-shelled turtles, pears, and persimmons.

How can we utilize the sour taste of food for dietetic health preservation?

The sour taste has astringent properties. Sour medicinals have the ability to constrict and bind, producing the effects such as stopping diarrhea, reducing sweating, astringing semen, reducing urine output, stopping abnormal vaginal discharge, and controlling bleeding. They can also constrict lung qi to alleviate coughing and calm the mind.

Sour-tasting medicinals can also generate body fluids. The famous story from the Three Kingdoms Period, "quenching thirst by looking at plums", demonstrates the ability of sour taste to generate body fluids. During scorching summer days, excessive sweating can lead to thirst and reduced urine output. In such cases, people often consume sour plum soup, which helps generate body fluids, stimulate appetite, relieve heat, quench thirst, relieve vexation and calm the mind.

sour-tasting medicinals can be used for symptoms such as dry mouth, lack of appetite, red tongue with little coating, or tongue peeling due to deficiency of stomach yin; spasms, and difficulty in flexing and extending the limbs due to consumption of body fluids and lack of nourishment in tendons and vessels; a weak constitution with excessive sweating, lung deficiency with chronic cough, chronic diarrhea, spermatorrhea, frequent urination, enuresis, and excessive vaginal bleeding. However, since most sour-tasting substances have astringent properties, they should be used with caution for conditions that have not fully resolved.

Sour-tasting foods include hawthorn, dried plums, papaya, pomegranate, apples, strawberries, etc. However, excessive consumption of sour-tasting foods can have certain side effects. As mentioned in the Tang Dynasty's *Materia Medica for Dietetic Therapy* that prolonged consumption of pomegranate can damage teeth, and excessive consumption of red bayberry can damage teeth and tendons. Therefore, moderation is key when consuming sour-tasting foods.

How can we utilize the bitter taste of food for dietetic health preservation?

The bitter taste has the ability to purge, dry, and strengthen, i.e. clearing heat, purging rebellious qi, promoting bowel movements, drying dampness, and nourishing yin (clearing heat while preserving yin). Generally, bitter-tasting medicinal substances are used for conditions related to heat and fire, coughing, vomiting, constipation, dampness, and excessive yang due to yin deficiency. However, bitter and dry substances can damage yin and fluids, so they should not be used for those who have insufficient yin. As bitter and cold substances are prone to damage the spleen and stomach yang qi, excessive dosage or prolonged use can lead to deficiency of spleen and stomach yang, loss of appetite, and loose stools. Therefore, those with a deficient spleen should also use bitter-tasting substances with caution.

Bitter-tasting foods include almonds, citron, daylily, Chinese wolfberry, balsam pear, Chinese lettuce, dandelion, artichoke, celery, etc. In recent years, more and more people are embracing a natural lifestyle and enjoying wild vegetables, most of which have a bitter taste. These bitter vegetables can clear heat and stimulate appetite, making them very beneficial for individuals prone to internal heat.

Tea has been consumed by Chinese people for thousands of years. Tea, which has a bitter taste, is considered cool in nature and has many benefits such as clearing the head and eyes, downbearing qi and pomoting digestion, and promoting bowel movements. In ancient times, tea was used to treat diarrhea, taking advantage of its ability to dry dampness and promote urination. However, excessive consumption of bitter-tasting foods can be harmful to the stomach, especially for those with a cold constitution.

How can we utilize the sweet taste of food for dietetic health preservation?

The sweet taste has the ability to nourish and moderate. Foods with a sweet taste have the effects of nourishing and moderating the body. In daily life, most staple foods have a sweet taste. TCM believes that the sweet taste enters the spleen and stomach, and sweet-tasting foods such as Chinese yam, jujubes, lotus seeds, barley, and white kidney beans can be used to nourish the spleen and stomach. Many commonly used prescriptions for nourishing the spleen and stomach, such as Shenling Baizhu San and Zisheng Wan, contain medicinal substances with a sweet taste. However, excessive intake of sweet-tasting foods can cause bloating and a sense of fullness, leading to loss of appetite.

How can we utilize the pungent taste of food for dietetic health preservation?

The pungent taste has the ability to disperse and promote circulation. It can promote qi circulation, invigorate the stomach, dispel cold, and activate blood circulation. There are many foods with a pungent taste, such as ginger, scallions, leeks, alcohol, coriander, peppers, Sichuan peppercorns, cinnamon, onions, fennel, and radish. pungent-tasting foods are generally hot in nature. It is a common practice to drink ginger soup when the abdomen feels cold to stimulate digestion and invigorate the stomach. When early signs of an external pathogen invasion appear, drinking scallion soup can help expel the pathogen and dispel cold. After childbirth, women often consume rice wine and brown sugar to dispel cold, promote qi circulation, and activate blood circulation. In regions with high humidity, such as Sichuan and Chongqing, residents tend to consume spicy foods like chili peppers and Sichuan peppercorns, which can effectively expel and resist dampness.

How can we utilize the salty taste of food for dietetic health preservation?

The salty taste has the ability to promote downward movement and soften hardness. It has the effects of promoting bowel movements, softening hard masses, and resolving accumulations. Generally, medicinal substances with a salty taste are used to treat constipation, phlegmatic nodules, goiter, abdominal masses, etc.

In addition, *Basic Questions–Xuanming Wuqi* also mentions the concept of "salty taste damaging the blood". The kidney pertains to water, and salty taste enters the kidney. The heart pertains to fire and governs blood. When salty taste enters the blood, it means that water overcomes fire. Medicinal substances such as Daqingye (Isatidis Folium), Xuanshen (Scrophulariae Radix), Zicao (Arnebiae Radix), Qingdai (Indigo Naturalis) and Baiwei (Cynanchi Atrati Radix et Rhizoma) all have a salty taste and can clear heat, cool the blood, and detoxify. In *Basic Questions–Zhizhenyao Dalun* it is also mentioned: "The five tastes enter the stomach, each has its preferred target...salty taste first enters the kidney." Therefore, many salty-tasting medicinal substances that enter the kidney meridian have good effects on kidney tonification. Some examples include Haigoushen (Callorhini Testes et Penis), and Gejie (Gecko). To enhance the tonifying effect on the kidney and guide medicinal substances to the kidney, some medicinal substances such as Zhimu (Anemarrhenae Rhizoma), Huangbo (Phellodendri Chinensis Cortex), and Duzhong (Eucommiae Cortex) are processed using saltwater.

How does Huangdi Neijing guide the combination of grain, fruit, vegetables and meat?

As early as more than 2, 000 years ago, *Basic Questions–Zangqi Fashi Lun* pointed out: "Five grains are used for nourishment, five fruits facilitate the nourishment, five livestock are used for tonification, and five vegetables are used for supplement. If they are taken in accordance with their qi and flavors, the essence and qi can be supplemented." It comprehensively summarized that grain, meat, vegetables and fruits are the main components of a diet, and at the same time, explained the law of formulating a diet, with grain as the staple food, meat as non-staple food, vegetables as the supplementary food and fruit as the auxiliary food.

What are the functions of commonly seen grains?

Grains have been the main staple food source of Chinese people since ancient times, and Zheng Xuan noted in *Rites of Zhou* that "grains" refers to "ma, shu, ji, mai and dou". The common characteristics of all kinds of grains are mild in nature, and sweet in flavor. Sweet flavor enters the spleen first, so long-term consumption of these staple foods can play an important role in recuperating spleen and stomach. Different kinds of grains have different properties. Sun Simiao, a famous health preservation expert in the Tang Dynasty, described the following several kinds of grains in detail in *Essential Recipes for Emergent Use Worth A Thousand Gold*.

Japonica rice (rice) tastes pungent, bitter and neutral and is non-toxic. It is used for polydipsia and diarrhea. It can calm stomach qi, promote muscle growth and warm the middle jiao.

Glutinous rice tastes bitter and warm and is non-toxic. It can warm the middle jiao and enable people to eat. It is hot in nature, so people will experience hard stool after taking it.

Stocked rice tastes salty and sour, is slightly cold in nature and is non-toxic. It can relieve irritability and heat, regulate digestion and relieve diarrhea.

Wheat tastes sweet, is slightly cold in nature and is non-toxic. It can nourish liver qi, remove guest heat, stop polydipsia and dryness in the throat, facilitate urination, and stop metrostaxis and hematemesis.

Buckwheat tastes sour, is slightly cold in nature and is non-toxic. It is hard to digest, and it can stir strong heat and wind. Its raw leaves can stir itchy wind, which makes people itch. Huangdi said that if it is made into noodles to be eaten with hot pork and mutton, the hot wind will be stirred within no more than 8 to 9 meals, which makes people's eyebrows fall off and grow again, but the eyebrow still little. In the north of Jingbin (now Bin County, Shaanxi Province), many people suffer from this disease.

Coix seed tastes sweet, is warm in nature and is non-toxic. It is used to treat tendon spasms, difficulty in flexing and extending, and long-term wind-dampness arthralgia with descending qi.

Soybean has a sweet taste, neutral and cool properties, and is non-toxic. When pounded into a paste and mixed with pure vinegar, it can be applied externally to treat various toxic swellings and alleviate pain. When it is boiled for juice and taken cold, it can eliminate ghost toxins, reduce edema, clear stomach heat, dispel wind-dampness, treat injuries and urinary disorders, remove blood stasis, disperse cold accumulations in the internal organs, counteract the toxic effects of aconitum, and neutralize the toxic effects of various drugs.

Red bean is neutral and cold in nature, sweet and salty in taste. It can relieve edema, expel pus and blood. But it cannot be taken for a long time, which can make people dry.

Mung bean tastes sweet and salty, warm, neutral and astringent in nature, and is non-toxic. It is used to treat cold and heat conditions, heat-related disorders, and xiaoke. It can also stop diarrhea, promote urination, alleviate vomiting and sudden dysentery, and relieve lower abdominal distension and fullness.

Fermented soybean tastes bitter and sweet, cold and astringent in nature, and is non-toxic. It is mainly used for headaches due to typhoid fever, alternate attacks of chill and fever, expelling miasma and poisons, irritability and distension, consumptive asthma, pain and cold in the feet, and killing various toxins.

What are the functions of commonly seen vegetables?

Wax gourd is sweet, tasteless and slightly cold with the effects of benefiting qi for promoting production of fluid, clearing heat and promoting diuresis.

Cucumber is sweet and cold with the effects of clearing heat and quenching thirst, promoting diuresis and removing toxicity.

Pumpkin is sweet and warm with the effects of invigorating spleen-stomach and replenishing qi, promoting diuresis and removing toxicity, and killing insects.

Celery leaves are bitter and slightly cold, with the effects of clearing heat and promoting diuresis, and lowering blood pressure and lipid.

Chinese chives are pungent and warm with the effects of warming yang and tonifying deficiency, promoting qi and regulating blood.

Tomato is sweet, sour, and slightly cold, with the effects of invigorating the spleen and promoting digestion, promoting production of fluid and quenching thirst, clearing heat and inducing diuresis, cooling blood and calming the liver.

Carrot is sweet and neutral with the effects of benefiting qi and blood, invigoratin the stomach and promoting digestion, improving eyesight and nourishing the liver.

Radish is pungent and cold with the effects of widening the middle jiao and lowering qi, dissipating phlegm and resolving food retention, clearing heat and removing toxicity, cooling blood and promoting production of fluid.

Eggplant is sweet and cold with the effects of clearing heat and harmonizing blood, dispelling blood stasis and reducing swelling.

Bamboo shoots are bitter and slightly cold with the effects of benefiting the five zang viscera, dredging meridians, strengthening bones and tendons, widening chest and benefiting qi.

Potato is sweet and neutral with the effects of invigorating spleen and qi, harmonizing the stomach and regulating middle jiao.

Lotus root is sweet and cold with the effects of the spleen and promoting appetite, moistening the lung and promoting production of fluid, cooling blood and clearing heat.

Kelp is salty and cold with the effects of eliminating phlegm and softening hard mass, clearing heat and promoting diuresis.

Mushrooms are sweet and neutral with the effects of invigorating qi and spleen, harmonizing the stomach and benefiting the kidney.

Agaric is sweet and neutral with the effects of invigorating qi and nourishing the brain, moistening the lung and promoting the production of fluid, stopping bleeding and cooling blood.

Chili is pungent and hot with the effects of warming the middle jiao and dispelling cold, promoting appetite and digestion, removing dampness and promoting sweating.

Garlic is pungent and warm with the effects of warming the middle jiao and dispelling cold, activating qi and resolving food retention, removing toxicity and killing insects.

Green onions are pungent and warm with the effects of relieving superficies and dispelling cold, activating yang and unblocking stuffy orifices.

What are the functions of commonly seen fruits?

Watermelon is sweet and cold in nature with the effects of clearing heat and summer heat, promoting production of fluid and inducing diuresis.

Peach is sweet, sour and warm and has the effects of invigorating qi and promoting production of fluid, promoting blood circulation and resolving food retention, and moistening intestines for relaxing bowels.

Pears are sweet, cold and slightly sour and have the effects of nourishing yin and promoting the production of fluid, moistening the lung and relieving cough, clearing heat and dissipating phlegm.

Plum is sweet, sour and neutral, and has the effects of clearing heat and promoting production of fluid, promoting diuresis and removing blood stasis.

Apricot is sour, sweet and warm and has the effects of promoting production of fluid and quenching thirst, moistening the lung and relieving dyspnea.

Chestnuts are sweet and warm and have the effects of tonifying bones and tendons, invigorating the spleen and benefiting qi, promoting blood circulation and stopping bleeding.

What are the functions of commonly seen meat products?

Pork is sweet, salty and neutral and has the effects of invigorating qi and nourishing blood, nourishing yin and moistening dryness, which can "enrich the body, nourish the skin, moisten the stomach and produce fluid". However, eating too much pork will cause production of phlegm and dampness, stirring wind and helping heat.

Beef is sweet, neutral and slightly warm, and has the effects of tonifying the spleen and benefiting qi, nourishing essence and blood, and strengthening the bones and tendons.

Mutton is sweet and warm and has the effects of invigorating qi and nourishing blood, warming kidney and dispelling cold.

Mutton, venison and rooster are relatively warm in nature and are suitable to be eaten in winter.

Hens are neutral in nature and are mostly used for parturients and blood loss patients.

Duck meat is cold in nature and can tonify deficiency and eliminate heat.

Section 4
Medicated Diet for Health Preservation

What are the ingredients of medicated diet?

The ingredients of medicated diet mainly refer to the food and traditional Chinese medicinals needed for dietetic health preservation. Generally, traditional Chinese medicinals are mostly tonic, and there are various kinds of food, including animals, plants, eggs and so on.

Traditional Chinese medicinals commonly used for nourishing qi, blood, yin and yang include: Renshen (Ginseng Radix et Rhizoma), Dangshen (Codonopsis Radix), Huangqi (Astragali Radix), Baizhu (Atractylodis Macrocephalae Rhizoma), Huaishanyao (Dioscoreae Rhizoma), Fuling (Poria), Danggui (Angelicae Sinensis Radix), Ejiao (Asini Corii Colla), Baishao (Paeoniae Radix Alba), Shudihuang (Rehmanniae Radix Praeparata), Taoren (Persicae Semen), Gouqizi (Lycii Fructus), Chuanbeimu (Fritillariae Cirrhosae Bulbus), Tiandong (Asparagi Radix), Baihe (Lilii Bulbus), Danzhuye (Lophatheri Herba), Maidong (Ophiopogonis Radix), Shashen (Glehniae Radix), Dongchongxiacao (Cordyceps), Ganjiang (Zingiberis Rhizoma), Roucongrong (Cistanches Herba), Lingzhi (Ganoderma), etc.

Common foods for nourishing qi, blood, yin and yang include: chicken, duck meat, fish, rabbit meat, mutton, sea cucumber, beef, pork liver, radish, bird's nest, soft-shelled turtle, wheat, mung bean, pigeon eggs, eggs, watermelon, pears, pork stomach, pork elbow, venison and so on.

Traditional Chinese medicinals commonly used for nourishing the heart, liver, spleen, lung and kidney include: Longyanrou (Longan Arillus), Suanzaoren (Ziziphi Spinosae Semen), Dangshen (Codonopsis Radix), Danggui (Angelicae Sinensis Radix), Baiziren (Platycladi Semen), Baihe (Lilii Bulbus), Gouqizi (Lycii Fructus), Juhua (Chrysanthemi Flos), Muzei (Equiseti Hiemalis Herba), mulberry, Baishao (Paeoniae Radix Alba), Huaishanyao (Dioscoreae Rhizoma), Sharen (Amomi Fructus), Doukou (Amomi Rotundus Fructus), Lianzi (Nelumbinis Semen), Dazao (Jujubae Fructus), Shanzha (Crataegi Fructus), Shenqu (Massa Medicata Fermentata), Baizhu (Atractylodis Macrocephalae Rhizoma), Baibiandou (Lablab Semen Album), Qianshi (Euryales Semen), Maidong

(Ophiopogonis Radix), Shashen (Glehniae Radix), Dongchongxiacao (Cordyceps), Chuanbeimu (Fritillariae Cirrhosae Bulbus), Yinxing (Ginkgo Folium), Hetaoren (Juglandis Semen), Shanzhuyu (Corni Fructus), Shudihuang (Rehmanniae Radix Praeparata), Tusizi (Cuscutae Semen), Gouji (Cibotii Rhizoma), etc.

Foods commonly used for nourishing the heart, liver, spleen, lung and kidney include: animal meat, heart, liver, stomach, kidney, penis, brain marrow, lung, etc.

Traditional Chinese medicinals commonly used for nourishing tendons, bones, skin, hair and teeth include: Duzhong (Eucommiae Cortex), Buguzhi (Psoraleae Fructus), Lujiao (Cervi Cornu), Lurong (Cervi Cornu Pantotrichum), Tusizi (Cuscutae Semen), Roucongrong (Cistanches Herba), Xuduan (Dipsaci Radix), Wujiapi (Acanthopanacis Cortex), Heshouwu (Polygoni Multiflori Radix), Hetaoren (Juglandis Semen), Dazao (Jujubae Fructus), Huaishanyao (Dioscoreae Rhizoma), Lianzi (Nelumbinis Semen), Heizhima (Sesami Semen Nigrum), mulberry, Gouqizi (Lycii Fructus), etc.

Foods commonly used for nourishing tendons, bones, skin, hair and teeth include: animal bones, kidney, tendon, meat, tail, bird's nest, eggs, rock sugar, honey, peanuts, etc.

What are the types and processing methods of medicated diet?

The production and application of traditional Chinese medicated diet can be considered not only a science but also an art. medicated diet comes in various forms, including soup, thick soup, porridge, paste, cakes, rolls, pot stickers, steamed buns, jelly, soup balls, pastry, etc. The basic processing methods include steaming, pan-frying, boiling, stewing, braising, simmering, cooking, stir-frying, deep-frying, baking, etc.

What are the classifications of medicated diet?

Generally speaking, according to the function of medicated diet, it can be divided into yin-nourishing, yang-strengthening, qi-invigorating, blood-replenishing, heart-nourishing for tranquilization, lung-tonifying, liver-nourishing and eyesight-improving, kidney- and essence-tonifying, spleen-invigorating and appetite-promoting, tendons- and bones-strengthening, skin-moistening, five zang viscera-harmonizing, hair-blackening and teeth-fixing, etc.

What are the commonly used medicinals and foods for the yin-nourishing medicated diet? What are their functions?

The yin-nourishing medicated diet is cooked by yin-nourishing medicinals, accompanied by food.

Traditional Chinese medicinals commonly used in the yin-nourishing medicated diet include Shengdihuang (Rehmanniae Radix), Huangjing (Polygonati Rhizoma), mulberry, Nüzhenzi (Ligustri Lucidi Fructus), Gouqizi (Lycii Fructus), Xuanshen (Scrophulariae Radix), Shudihuang (Rehmanniae Radix Praeparata), Tiandong (Asparagi Radix), Maidong (Ophiopogonis Radix), Shashen (Glehniae Radix), and Yuzhu (Polygonati Odorati Rhizoma). The main foods used are soft-shelled turtle, turtle, bird's nest, tremella and sea cucumber.

The functions of the yin-nourishing medicated diet include nourishing yin and increasing fluid, promoting production of fluid and quenching thirst, clearing heat and relieving dysphoria. It is suitable for thin limbs, haggard face, dry mouth and throat, sleeplessness caused by deficient dysphoria, even hectic fever and night sweating, choking cough without expectoration, hectic cheek, nocturnal emission and night emission, sore waist and back, caused by constitutional yin fluid insufficiency.

Yin-nourishing medicated diet is sweet, cold and greasy, which is not suitable for those with weak spleen and stomach, internal blockade of phlegm and dampness, abdominal distention and loose stool, and for those with exogenous diseases.

Examples of yin-nourishing medicated diet

Shengdihuang Chicken (from *Key to Diet*)

Composition: Shengdihuang (Rehmanniae Radix) 250 g, maltose 150 g, black-bone chicken 1 piece.
Making method: Use the above ingredients. Remove the feathers and internal organs of the chicken first, and wash it clean. Cut Shengdihuang (Rehmanniae Radix) intro slices and mix well with maltose, then put it in the belly of the

chicken. Put the chicken in a container, add some water, then place the contrainer in a steamer and steam over high heat until fully cooked.

Function: Nourishing yin and tonifying the kidney. It is suitable for backache, bone marrow deficiency, inability to stand for a long time, heavy body, lack of qi, night sweating, reduced appetite, and repeated vomiting.

Huangjing Stewed with Lean Pork (from folk recipe)

Composition: Huangjing (Polygonati Rhizoma) 50 g, lean pork 200 g, proper amount of onion, ginger, salt, and cooking wine.

Making method: Huangjing (Polygonati Rhizoma) and lean pork are cleaned and cut into pieces with a length of 3 cm and a width of 1.5 cm, put them into a tile pot (casserole), then add proper amount of water, onion, ginger, salt and cooking wine, and simmer over water.

Function: Nourishing spleen yin and benefiting the heart and lung. It is suitable for daily recuperation of yin deficiency constitution, as well as reduced appetite and insomnia caused by yin and blood deficiency of the heart and spleen.

Mulberry Mash (from *Indentification of Materia Medica*)

Composition: Fresh mulberries 1 000 g, glutinous rice 500 g, a proper amount of distiller's yeast.

Making method: Clean fresh mulberries and mash them into juice (or decoct 300 g of dry products and remove slag), then cook the medicinal juice together with 500 g of glutinous rice to make dry rice, mix it with proper amount of distiller's yeast when cold, ferment them into fermented wine, and eat it in appropriate amount with meal every day.

Function: Replenishing blood and kidney, improving hearing and eyesight. It is suitable for consumptive thirst, constipation, tinnitus, dark eyes, cervical scrofula and joint disorders due to yin deficiency of the liver and kidney.

What are the commonly used medicinals and foods for the yang-strengthening medicated diet? What are their functions?

The yang-strengthening medicated diet is made with yang-strengthening medicinals, accompanied by food.

Traditional Chinese medicinals often used in the yang-strengthening medicated diet include Lujiao (Cervi Cornu), Ganjiang (Zingiberis Rhizoma), bull penis, animal kidneys and so on. The selected foods are mutton, venison and so on.

The functions of the yang-strengthening medicated diet are: strengthening yang and tonifying the kidney, warming the interior and dispelling cold, benefiting essence and enriching blood. It is suitable for impotence, spermatorrhea, white turbidity, leukorrhea, soreness of waist and knees, fear of cold, cold limbs, reduced appetite and diarrhea.

The yang-strengthening medicated diet is warm and dry, and is not suitable for heat diseases, syndrome of endogenous heat due to yin deficiency, carbuncle and abscess, sore and toxin, etc. This kind of medicated diet is recommended in winter.

Examples of yang-strengthening medicated diet

Lujiao Porridge (from *Quxian Huoren Fang*)

Composition: Lujiao (Cervi Cornu) powder 5–10 g, japonica rice 30–60 g, a little salt.

Making method: Cook porridge with japonica rice first, add Lujiao (Cervi Cornu) powder in the boiling rice soup, add a little salt, and cook them into porridge.

Function: Tonifying kidney yang, benefiting essence and blood, and strengthening bones and tendons. It is suitable for fear of cold, cold body, soreness of waist and knees, impotence, premature ejaculation, infertility and mental fatigue due to deficiency of kidney yang, essence and blood; children with hypoplasia, bone softness and retardation in walking, and failure of closure of fontanel; metrorrhagia and metrostaxis, and leukorrhea in women; inner collapse of yin carbuncle and abscess, sores and ulcerations that fail to heal for a long time. It is recommended to be taken in winter. It is not suitable for people with internal heat, hyperactivity of yang due to yin deficiency, or exogenous fever caused by yang deficiency.

What are the commonly used medicinals and foods in the qi-invigorating medicated diet? What are their functions?

The qi-invigorating medicated diet is made with qi-invigorating traditional Chinese medicinals and spleen-tonifying and stomach-invigorating food.

Traditional Chinese medicinals used for the qi-invigorating medicated diet include Renshen (Ginseng Radix et Rhizoma), Dangshen (Codonopsis Radix), Huangqi (Astragali Radix), Huaishanyao (Dioscoreae Rhizoma), etc. The selected foods are chicken, fish, pork and so on.

The functions of the qi-invigorating medicated diet are: tonifying qi and supplementing middle jiao, strengthening the spleen and stomach. It is suitable for shortness of breath, cough and asthma, fatigue, poor appetite due to deficiency of lung and spleen-qi, and it is also suitable for the elderly with weak constitution, rectal prolapse due to long-term disease and other diseases.

Qi-invigorating medicated diet is tonic, but it should not be eaten too much at one time. It should be taken in small amounts for a long time; people with weak constitution need to prevent the condition of being "too weak to be tonified". Also, it is not suitable for excess syndrome, heat syndrome and the early stage of exogenous diseases.

Examples of qi-invigorating medicated diet

Steamed Shenqi Chicken (from *Food Recuperation Method for Common Chronic Diseases*)

Composition: Dangshen (Codonopsis Radix) 30 g, honey-fried Huangqi (Astragali Radix) 60 g, a hen (1 000–1 500 g), fine salt, yellow wine.

Making method: Dangshen (Codonopsis Radix) is rinsed and cut into slices, then soak it with a spoonful of yellow wine. Remove the feathers of the hen, wash it and cut it into small pieces. Put the chicken, Dangshen (Codonopsis Radix) and honey-fried Huangqi (Astragali Radix) in a bowl, add a spoonful of fine salt, and a spoonful of yellow wine, and steam it for 3 hours until the chicken is cooked.

Function: Invigorating qi and stomach, tonifying deficiency for relieving desertion. It is suitable for those with weak constitution, fear of cold, the elderly with rectal prolapse due to qi deficiency, and polyphagia with the tendency to be hungry.

Milk Porridge (from *Health and Longevity*)

Composition: Milk 500 ml, a proper amount of rice.

Making method: Wash the rice and cook it in a pot. When it is half cooked, add milk and cook it thoroughly.

Function: Invigorating qi and tonifying deficiency. It is suitable for qi deficiency of the spleen and stomach and weak constitution.

What are the commonly used medicinals and foods in the blood-replenishing medicated diet? What are their functions?

The blood-replenishing medicated diet is made by blood-replenishing traditional Chinese medicinals and foods.

Commonly used traditional Chinese medicinals are: Danggui (Angelicae Sinensis Radix), Shudihuang (Rehmanniae Radix Praeparata), Dangshen (Codonopsis Radix), Huangqi (Astragali Radix), Ejiao (Asini Corii Colla), Baishao (Paeoniae Radix Alba), Chuanxiong (Chuanxiong Rhizoma), Tianqi (Notoginseng Radix et Rhizoma), Gouqizi (Lycii Fructus), Jixueteng (Spatholobi Caulis). The selected foods mainly include mutton, beef, chicken, duck and so on.

The functions of the blood-replenishing medicated diet are replenishing and nourishing blood, which is suitable for pale complexion, spiritlessness and fatigue, vertigo and dizziness, palpitation, insomnia and menstrual disorder caused by blood deficiency. Most of these medicated diets are greasy products, so they are not suitable for those with excess heat, phlegm and dampness flatulence and exogenous fever.

Examples of blood-replenishing medicated diet

Stewed Chicken with Tianqi (from *Dietetic Health Preservation Recipe*)

Composition: Hen 1300 g, Tianqi (Notoginseng Radix et Rhizoma) 15 g, ginger 20 g, green onion 30 g, refined salt 10 g, Shaoxing wine 30 g.

Making method: Grind Tianqi (Notoginseng Radix et Rhizoma) into powder. Wash the hen, ginger and green onion. Add clean water and chicken in a casserole, boil over a strong fire, skim off the blood foam after boiling, and add ginger, green onion and Shaoxing wine. Use mild fire to stew them until they become soft. Add Tianqi (Notoginseng Radix et Rhizoma) powder, and refined salt for seasoning.

Function: Replenishing blood and tonifying qi, promoting blood circulation and dispelling blood stasis. It is suitable for postpartum women with deficiency of qi and blood, pain in the lower abdomen, prolonged lochiorrhea, and hemoptysis caused by lung consumption.

Ejiao Baipi Porridge (from *Dietetic Health Preservation Recipe*)

Composition: Ejiao (Asini Corii Colla) 15 g, Sangbaipi (Mori Cortex) 15 g, glutinous rice 100 g, brown sugar 8 g.

Making method: Wash Sangbaipi (Mori Cortex), put it in a casserole and decoct it into juice twice. Wash glutinous rice, and put it in a pot. Add clear water and boil it for 10 minutes, and then pour the medicinal juice and Ejiao (Asini Corii Colla). Add brown sugar and cook porridge out of them.

Function: Nourishing yin and replenishing blood, moistening dryness and clearing lung. It is suitable for hemoptysis due to chronic cough, hematochezia, hypomenorrhea, metrorrhagia and metrostaxis and threatened miscarriage caused by deficiency of yin and blood, deficiency of lung yin and fluid injury.

Section 5
Dietary Recommendations and Restrictions

What is the appropriate amount of food intake?

Huangdi Neijing emphasized "eating and drinking moderately", mainly indicating that a diet with a proper amount and schedule should be set. Not eating too much is the first principle of ancient dietetic health preservation. Because "doubled amount of diet will do harm to spleen and stomach", over-satiety is an important cause of spleen and stomach damage. *General Treatise on Causes and Manifestations of All Diseases* in the Sui Dynasty pointed out that besides dysphoria and sleeplessness, over-satiety can easily cause amassment and accumulation that are hard to resolute, pain in the upper abdominal mass, inflexibility of limbs and joints, darkish complexion and macula on the face, low back pain and edema. And in severe cases, over-satiety can also result in blockage of all vessels, leading to impairment of life span. The correct amount of food intake varies from person to person. *Essential Recipes for Emergent Use Worth a Thousand Gold* suggests that the correct method is to "speak cautiously and control one's diet. Therefore, those who are good at nurturing their health should eat when they are slightly hungry and drink when they are slightly thirsty. They should have several small meals with moderate appetite, avoiding overeating, as it hampers digestion. It is advisable to always aim for a state of being satisfied but not bloated, and hungry but not empty. Excessive fullness harms the lung, while hunger harms the qi...Therefore, it is recommended to adopt a light diet, chew food thoroughly, and ensure that digested rice enters the stomach rather than alcohol". It emphasizes the need for moderation and regularity in diet, advises against consuming too much in one meal, and suggests maintaining a state of satiety without feeling overly full, and hunger without feeling empty. Su Dongpo, a famous scholar in the Song Dynasty, had a famous saying of "three nourishments": "Be calm for the nourishment of good will, widen the stomach for the nourishment of qi, and reflect the responsibility for the nourishment of wealth." Being calm and reflecting the responsibility are the experience of life, while widening the stomach means that the stomach is in a state of relaxation and smoothness, and the stomach cannot be stuffed too full.

What suggestions did the ancients give on eating time?

The ancients had the most precepts on dinner for the three meals of the day. At the end of the Tang Dynasty, *Yixin Fang* set up a special section of "Food Prohibited at Night", which put forward that "don't be too full in the evening. In this way, you stay away from diseases". If people are too full at night and remain inactive, it is difficult for them to digest and will lead to diseases. Shi Chengjin in the Qing Dynasty put forward the best time for dinner: "Lunch time should be before noon, and dinner time should be before sunset. In a word, people should wait for an hour after the meal, till the drink and food move downward. In this way, there will be no hidden danger." The ancients thought that it was inappropriate to have dinner after seven o'clock.

What suggestions did the ancients give on eating speed?

Health Preservation for the Elderly quoted Huo Tuo's *Discussion on Diet and Foods* said that "food has three transformations: one is fire transformation, which refers to boiling the food with external fire; one is mouth transformation, which refers to chewing the food; one is abdomen transformation, which refers to digesting the food in the stomach". That is to say, when eating, people should chew slowly, and the eating speed should not be too fast. Especially for people with bad intestine and stomach functions and the elderly, digesting foodin theintestines and stomach themselves is already a heavy burden. Therefore, cooking food thoroughly and chewing it slowly are good ways to help with digestion. Shi Chengjin, a doctor in the Qing Dynasty, listed three major benefits of chewing slowly: "First, chewing slowly can help the essence of food nourish the five zang viscera; second, it is conducive to the digestion of spleen and stomach; third, in this way, people will not get choked."

What suggestions did the ancients give for the flavors of food?

The ancients advocated that diet should be tasteless, where "tasteless" has two meanings. One is plain, which corresponds to the greasy and surfeit flavor of food. The other is bland, which corresponds to the salty flavor. There are many discussions on the plain diet by the ancients. Since *Basic Questions*, the ancients have advocated plain diets and have been critical of overeating fish and meat with greasy and surfeit flavor. *Basic Questions* thinks that if normal people overeat "greasy and surfeit flavor", that is, overeating fatty food with heavy flavor, diseases of sores and ulcers will occur. And patients should pay more attention to the plain diet. For instance, "in the recovery process from heat disease, eating meat will result in a relapse, and even eating a large amount of meat will lead to some sequelae". Most doctors of later generations have inherited this view. For example, Sun Simiao in the Tang Dynasty said in *Essential Recipes for Emergent Use Worth A Thousand Gold* that "meals don't need heavy meat, because it will cause all kinds of diseases". In ancient times, it was late to advocate eating food of tasteless flavor, and the clear exposition can be seen in *The Secret of Longevity* in the Qing Dynasty: "Tasteless food is the most beneficial, and each of the five flavors hurts...Among the five flavors, salty taste can coagulate blood and stagnate qi, which hurts people even more." It is believed that overeating salty flavor can make the face haggard and stagnate blood vessels.

What are the ancient dietetic contraindications?

Dietetic contraindications are also called "food contraindications", or "food taboos". The contents of ancient dietetic contraindications are extensive, including the contraindications of toxic substances, the contraindications of various special populations, the contraindications of various food collocations, the contraindications of patients and people who are taking medicines, etc. The earliest dietetic contraindications recorded in the *Book of Han–Yiwen Zhi* is *Shennong Huangdi Food Contraindications*. Before the Sui and Tang Dynasties, there were many books about dietetic contraindications, such as *Laozi's Classics of Food Contraindications, Shennong's Food Taboos*, and *Bianque's Food Contraindications*.

Toxic substances are the most important problem in early dietetic health preservation. Some of these items are toxic themselves, and some of their toxins are caused by pollution, long-term decomposition, or other factors. Zhang Zhongjing, a famous doctor in the Han Dynasty who was revered as a medical sage by the later world, attached "Treatment for Contraindications of Animals, Insects and Fish" and "Treatment for Contraindications of Fruits, Vegetables and Grains" in his works, summarizing the contraindications of animal and plant foods before the Han Dynasty, and he also listed many detoxifying methods for food poisoning.

In ancient times, there were many contraindications for eating animals. In *Health Preservation Food Taboos*, the rage of contraindications was expanded to the extent that all animals and plants with strange and unique shapes were considered to be unfavorable to the human body. For example, animals with huge claws couldn't be eaten, fish with inversed scales or gills couldn't be eaten, and fish who can open and close their eyes couldn't be eaten, and so on.

Contraindications of special populations are commonly known as "restrictions on mouth". Among the so-called special populations, most emphasis is put on children, pregnant and labored women, the elderly, and patients. TCM pays great attention to the diet of various special populations, and patients who take medicine should pay attention not to eat food that has the opposite nature of the medicine they take or is not conducive to the action of the medicine. In *Materia Medica for Dietetic Therapy* in the Tang Dynasty, it is recorded that "children should not be given fried beans. If they eat them with pork, most of them will die from qi stagnation". Children's spleen and stomach functions are not sound, and legumes are difficult to digest, especially fried beans. If they eat greasy pork after eating fried beans, although they will not develop to the extent that "most of them will die", it is undoubtedly not conducive to children's health. In ancient times, people were most particular about the dietetic contraindications of pregnant and labored women. The general principle is "cool before delivery and warm after delivery". Because women mostly eat the food of hot nature in the prenatal period, which is easy to cause threatened miscarriage, and result in diseases of sores, ulcers, furuncles and boils; in the puerperium, if women eat mostly food of cold nature, blood stasis will remain in the body, causing prolonged lochiorrhea and postpartum abdominal pain. Women in the lactation period should also pay attention to diet. Some foods may result in hypogalactia, such as sour pomegranate. Some foods may enter the infants' bodies through milk, causing corresponding adverse reactions in infants, commonly known as "passed-on milk".

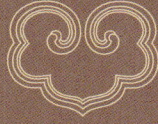

Chapter 6

Medicinal Health Preservation

Section 1

Overview of Medicinal Health Preservation

What is medicinal health preservation?

Medicinal health preservation employs Chinese medicinals either internally or externally under the guidance of TCM theories, to achieve a comprehensive adjustment of the body through their nutritive and regulating effects. This involves harmonizing qi and blood, balancing yin and yang, regulating organs, and ensuring the smooth flow of meridians to improve health and prolong life.

What are the characteristics of medicinal health preservation?

The classic *Huangdi Neijing* introduces the concept of "preventing disease before its onset". *Basic Questions–Siqi Tiaoshen Dalun* said: "Therefore, the wise do not treat the diseased but the undiseased, not the chaotic but the unchaotic. To treat a disease only after it manifests or to order only after chaos ensues is akin to digging a well when thirsty or forging a needle during a battle—surely too late." This highlights the profound significance of disease prevention and further elucidates the critical role of medicinal health preservation in both disease prevention and treatment. In summary, medicinal health preservation is characterized by the following three aspects:

First, prevention before onset. The occurrence of diseases is related to two aspects: the body's healthy energy (zhengqi) and pathogenic factors (xieqi). The role of medicinal health preservation also involves the joint action of these two aspects. Firstly, it involves nurturing the body and enhancing the body's healthy energy to resist pathogenic factors. As stated in *Suwen Yipian–Cifa Lun*: "When the body's healthy energy is maintained internally, pathogenic factors cannot interfere." For individuals with a weak constitution and insufficient healthy energy, taking appropriate tonifying medicinals can support healthy energy, strengthen the body, and prevent the occurrence of diseases. Secondly, it involves avoiding toxic influences and preventing the invasion of pathogenic factors. *Basic Questions–Shanggu Tianzhen Lun* mentions: "For external pathogenic factors and harmful winds, avoid them in a timely manner." In addition to enhancing healthy energy and boosting disease resistance, medicinal health preservation can also prevent the invasion of pathogenic factors. Using Guanzhong (Dryopteridis Crassirhizomatis Rhizoma), Banlangen (Isatidis Radix), and Daqingye (Isatidis Folium) to prevent influenza, Yinchen (Artemisiae Scopariae Herba) and Zhizi (Gardeniae Fructus) to prevent hepatitis, and Machixian (Portulacae Herba) to prevent bacterial dysentery have all achieved very good preventive and therapeutic effects.

Second, preventing progression in existing illness. If disease has already set in, early diagnosis and treatment are crucial. In *Basic Questions–Yinyang Yingxiang Dalun*, it is stated: "When pathogenic wind invades, it strikes swiftly like wind and rain. Therefore, a skilled healer treats the skin and hair, the next best treats the muscles and flesh, the next treats the tendons and vessels, the next treats the six fu organs, and the last treats the five zang organs. Treating the five zang organs is akin to being half alive and half dead." This illustrates that when external pathogens invade the body, if not diagnosed and treated promptly, the disease will progress from the exterior to the interior, worsening the condition. Therefore, early treatment is essential to prevent the disease from penetrating deeper and affecting the five zang organs, complicating the illness. In *Nan Jing– Seventy-seven Difficult Issues*, it is stated: "The superior healer treats before disease occurs, the average healer treats existing disease...To treat before disease means that upon observing a liver disorder, one knows it may transmit to the spleen, and thus strengthens the spleen's energy first to prevent it from being affected by the liver's disorder. This is called treating before disease. The average healer, seeing a liver disorder, does not understand transmission and focuses solely on treating the liver, thus it is called treating existing disease." This is the practical application of the principle of preventing disease transformation. According to the law of disease transmission, one should first secure the areas not yet affected by pathogens, preventing the spread and transmission of disease to protect the unaffected organs.

Third, prevention of recurrence. Post-disease recuperation should involve appropriate medicinal support to restore vital energy, ensure smooth circulation of qi and blood, and nourish the organs, so as to achieve the balance of yin and yang, preventing recurrence from pathogen. In the *Treatise on Cold Damage*, it is stated: "After the resolution of cold damage, for symptoms of weakness, fatigue, shortness of breath, and rebellious qi causing nausea, Zhuye Shigao Decoction is recommended." It suggests using Zhuye Shigao Decoction to manage emaciation, residual weakness, shortness of breath, fatigue and hectic low fever after febrile illness, which are caused by residual heat disturbing upward, This formula replenishes qi, promotes fliud production, and clears heat by its sweet and cold nature, thus clearing away residual pathogens and nourishing both qi and yin.

What is the principle of medicinal nourishment?

A key condition for health and longevity is a strong innate constitution and adequate acquired nutrition. Additionally, it requires a balance of yin and yang, harmony of qi and blood, and unobstructed meridians. The kidney is considered the foundation of innate endowment, while the spleen and stomach are the foundation of acquired nutrition. Therefore, medicinal nourishment often focuses on strengthening and protecting both the innate and acquired aspects, with an emphasis on the spleen and kidney. It also takes into account the five organs, qi and blood, and yin and yang. By enhancing the innate, regulating the spleen and stomach, harmonizing the five zang viscera, balancing yin and yang, harmonizing qi and blood, and ensuring smooth meridians, the goal is to nourish the body, promote longevity, prevent disease, and strengthen the body.

Section 2
Commonly Used
Traditional Chinese
Medicinals for
Health Preservation

How many traditional Chinese medicinals are known for their health-preserving functions?

According to one of the four great TCM classical texts, *Shennong's Classic of Materia Medica*: "There are 120 superior herbs, which govern nourishment and align with the heavens." "There are 120 middle herbs, which maintain nature and conform to humanity." "There are 125 inferior herbs, which treat diseases and correspond to the earth." Among the 365 herbs listed in the book, 165 herbs are noted for their effects on prolonging life, anti-aging, endurance enhancement, boosting qi, lightening the body, and increasing longevity. In the Ming Dynasty, Li Shizhen's *Compendium of Materia Medica* documented 1892 medicinal substances, 253 of which are recognized for their anti-aging and life-extending functions, including 89 longevity formulas. During the Qing Dynasty, the ruling class had a keen interest in elixirs purported to confer immortality, hence numerous such prescriptions were popular in the palace, such as Yishou Paste, Buyi Zisheng Pills, Juhua Yanling Paste, Bailin Pills, and Songling Taiping Chun Wine.

What are the commonly used medicinals for body nourishment and longevity?

Frequently used medicinals include Renshen (Ginseng Radix et Rhizoma), Lurong (Cervi Cornu Pantotrichum), Dongchongxiacao (Cordyceps), Ejiao (Asini Corii Colla), Gouqizi (Lycii Fructus), Shudihuang (Rehmanniae Radix Praeparata), Shengdihuang (Rehmanniae Radix), Roucongrong (Cistanches Herba), Bajitian (Morindae Officinalis Radix), Tusizi (Cuscutae Semen), Fuling (Poria), Niuxi (Achyranthis Bidentatae Radix), Tiandong (Asparagi Radix), Yuanzhi (Polygalae Radix), Duzhong (Eucommiae Cortex), Wuweizi (Schisandrae Chinensis Fructus), Baizhu (Atractylodis Macrocephalae Rhizoma), Changpu (Accri Tatarinowii Rhizoma), Danggui (Angelicae Sinensis Radix), Maidong (Ophiopogonis Radix), Shanzhuyu (Corni Fructus), Heshouwu (Polygoni Multiflori Radix), Buguzhi (Psoraleae Fructus), Shanyao (Dioscoreae Rhizoma), Huangqi (Astragali Radix),

Yiyiren (Coicis Semen), Longyanrou (Longan Arillus), Yuzhu (Polygonati Odorati Rhizoma), Huangjing (Polygonati Rhizoma), mulberry, Nüzhenzi (Ligustri Lucidi Fructus), Ciwujia (Acanthopanacis Senticosi Radix et Rhizoma Seu Caulis), Dangshen (Codonopsis Radix), Zaoren (Ziziphi Spinosae Semen), Gancao (Glycyrrhizae Radix et Rhizoma), Dazao (Jujubae Fructus), etc. Among these, those used for kidney nourishment and essence replenishment are most frequently used, followed by spleen-strengthening and qi-enhancing medicinals, and heart-soothing and mind-calming medicinals.

What are the qi-boosting traditional Chinese medicinals?

Qi-boosting medicinals are known for their invigorating effects, which enhance physical strength and are particularly suitable for conditions of qi deficiency, especially involving the lung and spleen. Here are some commonly used qi-boosting medicinals:

Renshen (Ginseng Radix et Rhizoma)

Originated from the root and rhizome of the *Panax ginseng*, a plant in the Araliaceae family. Mildly warm in nature, sweet and slightly bitter in taste, it enters the spleen and lung meridians. It significantly boosts primal qi, generates fluids to quench thirst, enhances mental function, and calms the spirit. Its primary components include ginsenosides and amino acids. It can treat symptoms like weakness, thirst with a desire for drink, dreaminess, poor sleep, spontaneous sweating, palpitations, vomiting, cold stomach pain, shortness of breath, chronic cough, and decreased libido.

Renshen (Ginseng Radix et Rhizoma) is classified by processing method and cultivation: wild ginseng, transplanted wild ginseng, cultivated ginseng, sun-dried ginseng, red ginseng (steamed and dried), and white ginseng (cooked and sugar-infused). Among these, wild ginseng from older plants is considered superior. Red ginseng has a stronger effect compared to the sun-dried, and white ginseng is milder. Ginseng, while highly valued as a tonic, should

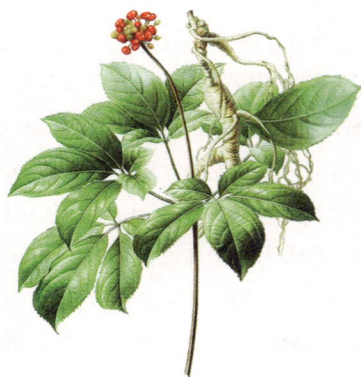

Renshen

not be overused, otherwise it can cause side effects like constipation, nosebleeds, bloating, insomnia, and irritability.

Huangqi (Astragali Radix)

Originated from the roots of *Astragalus membranaceus* or *Astragalus mongholicus*, it is warm, sweet, and associates with the spleen and lung meridians. It boosts qi, raises yang, strengthens the exterior to stop sweating, promotes healing of sores, and has diuretic and swelling-reducing effects. Honey-prepared astragalus is used to enhance qi boosting, while raw astragalus is preferred for stopping sweat, promoting diuresis, and healing sores. It can be used to address symptoms like weakness, spontaneous and night sweating, dizziness due to blood deficiency, chronic hepatitis, numb limbs, pain, edema with oliguria, and slow-healing sores.

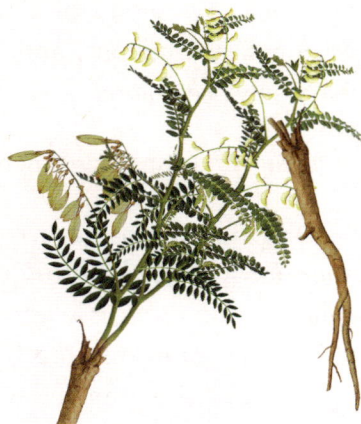

Huangqi

Baizhu (Atractylodis Macrocephalae Rhizoma)

The rhizome of *Atractylodes macrocephala*, belonging to the Asteraceae family, is warm and tastes both sweet and bitter. It enters the spleen and stomach meridians, with functions to strengthen the spleen, dry dampness, promote water metabolism, and stop sweating. It is a key herb for spleen strengthening and damp drying. Depending on the desired therapeutic effect, it is prepared differently: charred or fried for strengthening the spleen and stomach, earth-fried for stopping diarrhea and strengthening the spleen, and raw for promoting diuresis and stopping sweating.

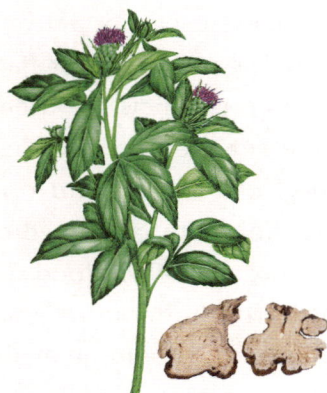

Baizhu

It is used to treat abdominal distention, poor appetite, spleen deficiency with loose stools, spontaneous and night sweating, diarrhea due to heat exhaustion, phlegm-fluid retention, drooling in children, etc.

What are the blood-nourishing traditional Chinese medicinals?

Blood-nourishing traditional Chinese medicinals primarily target blood deficiency. Symptoms of blood deficiency include pallor, pale lips and nails, dizziness, palpitations, and irregular menstruation in women. Here are some commonly used blood-nourishing herbs:

Danggui (Angelicae Sinensis Radix)

Originated from the root of the *Angelica sinensis*, belonging to the Apiaceae family. It is warm in nature with sweet, pungent, and bitter taste, and enters the heart, liver, lung, and spleen meridians. It is a key herb for treating blood sydnrome, and is known for nourishing blood, regulating menstruation, activating blood circulation to alleviate pain, and moistening the intestines to promote bowel movements. For nourishing blood, the main body of the root is used; for activating blood,

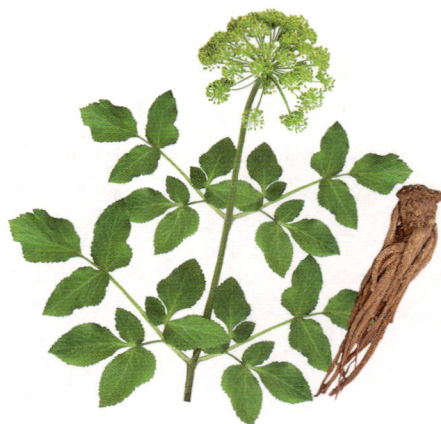

Danggui

the tail is preferred; for harmonizing blood, the whole root is utilized. The prepared products are used for nourishing blood and moistening intestines, while stir-fried product (especially fried with wine) is used to invigorate blood circulation and regulate menstruation. It is effective in treating conditions like combined deficiency of qi and blood, cold abdominal pain due to deficiency, blood deficiency with constipation, menstrual disorders, postpartum abdominal pain, chronic hepatitis, and chronic bronchitis. However, it should be avoided in cases of excessive dampness, diarrhea, or heavy menstrual bleeding.

Ejiao (Asini Corii Colla)

Made from the skin of donkeys, this gelatin is processed by soaking and removing hair, then boiling down into a solid form. It can be used directly or processed with clamshell powder or cattail pollen to form Ejiao pearls (clamshell for lung conditions, cattail for bleeding). Neutral in nature and sweet in taste, it enters the liver, lung, and kidney meridians. It is valued for its ability to nourish blood, stop bleeding, moisten dryness, and enrich yin. It is commonly used in winter tonics (with donkey-hide gelatin, rice wine, walnuts, black sesame, red dates, longan, etc.) and can also treat dizziness, palpitations, restlessness, insomnia, chronic dry cough, spitting blood, heavy menstrual flow, metrorrhagia and metrostaxis, etc. Being sweet and sticky, Ejiao nourishes and enriches the blood and is crucial for treating blood deficiency. However, caution is advised in cases of real heat or blood stasis, as premature use may lead to retained stasis. Raw Ejiao can be hard on the stomach, so those with weak spleen and stomach functions should use it cautiously.

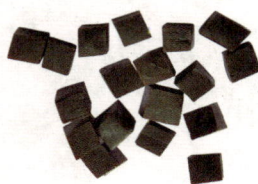

Ejiao

Shudihuang (Rehmanniae Radix Praeparata)

It is a processed product of Shengdihuang (Rehmanniae Radix). It is sweet and slightly warm, entering the heart, liver, and kidney meridians. It is renowned for nourishing blood, regulating menstruation, nourishing the kidney, and cultivating yin. It can treat symptoms due to qi and blood deficiency, insufficient essence and blood. Shudihuang can not only enrich yin

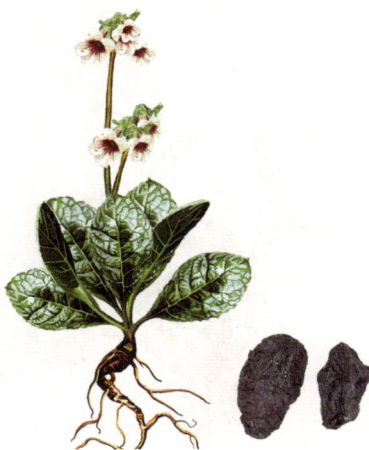

Shudihuang

and nourish blood but also generate essence and and marrows, and strengthen bones. It is a key herb used to nourish the liver and kidney. However, its sticky nature can hinder transportation and transformation of spleen and stomach, so it should be used with caution in individuals with weak digestion, excessive phlegm, or loose stools. To mitigate its rich and cloying nature, it is often prescribed with Sharen (Amomi Fructus) or aromatic medicinals with effect of invigorating the spleen.

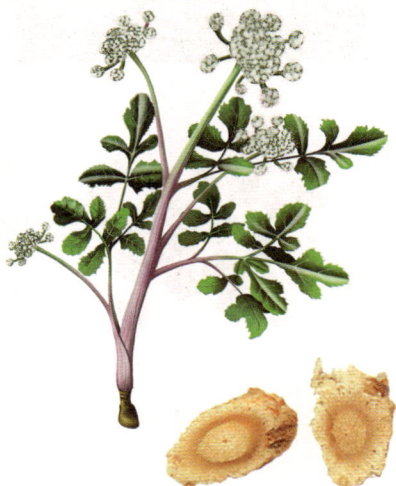

Beishashen

What are the yin-nourishing traditional Chinese medicinals?

Yin-nourishing traditional Chinese medicinals focus on enriching yin, increasing body fluids, and moisturizing dryness. They are particularly suitable for conditions marked by yin deficiency and fluid depletion. Here are some commonly used yin-nourishing herbs:

Beishashen (Glehniae Radix)

Originated from the root of the *Glehnia littoralis*, a plant in the Apiaceae family, it is slightly cool in nature with a sweet and slightly bitter taste, entering the lung and stomach meridians. It is effective in moistening the lung to stop coughs and enriching the stomach to generate fluids. It can be used to treat symptoms like thirst, dry tongue, laborious cough with bloody sputum, and dry cough due to yin deficiency. It is not suitable for those with cold-deficiency conditions.

Shihu (Dendrobii Caulis)

Originated from the stems of *Dendrobium* spp., belonging to Orchidaceae family, it is

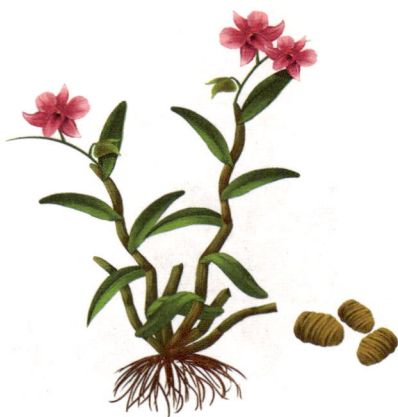

Shihu

cool in nature with a sweet taste, entering the lung, stomach, and kidney meridians. Known for its ability to nourish the stomach, generate fluids, enrich yin, and clear heat, it is a commonly used herb to nourish stomach yin. It can be used to treat conditions like dry mouth, thirst, chronic low-grade fever, dry cough without phlegm, and visual deterioration.

Guijia (Testudinis Carapax et Plastrum)

It comes from the carapace and plastron of turtles, belonging to the Testudinidae family. It is neutral in nature with sweet and salty flavors, and enters the kidney, heart, and liver meridians. It has the effects of nourishing yin, subduing yang, strengthening the kidney, fortifying bones, and stabilizing the essence to stop bleeding. It can be used to treat symptoms like palpitations due to fright, dizziness, excessive menstrual flow, and weak sinews and bones. Given its cold and salty nature, it should not be used by individuals with spleen and stomach cold-deficiency or those with unresolved external pathogenic factors.

What are the yang-nourishing traditional Chinese medicinals?

Yang-nourishing medicinals are primarily used for yang deficiency, which includes deficiencies of heart yang, spleen yang, and kidney yang. Since the kidney is considered the source of congenital constitution, yang-nourishing treatments often focus on strengthening kidney yang. These medicinals typically have effects of warming the kidney and strengthening yang, replenishing essence and marrows, and strengthening sinews and bones. Here are some commonly used yang-nourishing medicinals:

Lurong (Cervi Cornu Pantotrichum)

This is the hairy young horn of *Cervus nippon* or *Cervus elaphus* which has not yet calcified into bone. When it grows and sheds its velvet to become bony, it is known as deer horn, and the gelatin derived from boiling the horn is called deer horn glue. Lurong is warm in nature with sweet and salty flavors, entering

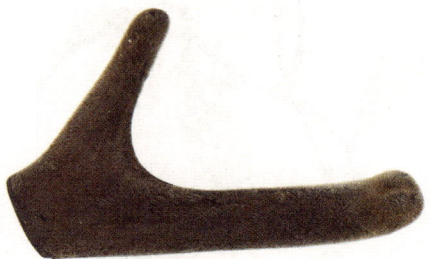

Lurong

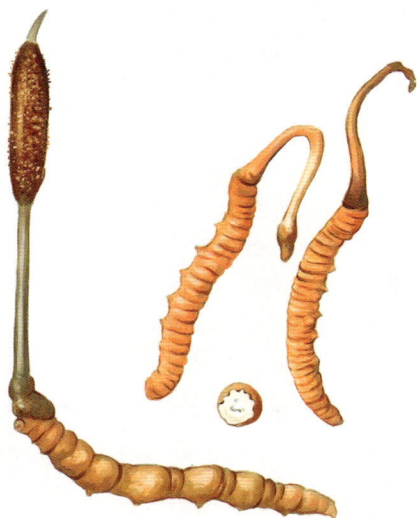

Dongchongxiacao

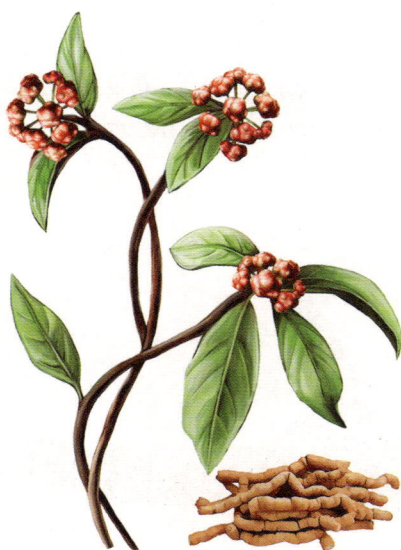

Bajitian

the liver and kidney meridians. It has the efficacy of tonifying kidney yang, enriching the blood and essence, and strengthening sinews and bones. It can be used to treat conditions such as general debility, cardiac weakness, deficiency of kidney essence, poor growth in children, leukorrhea, menorrhagia and metrostaxis, and anemia.

Dongchongxiacao (Cordyceps)

This is a complex of the stroma of the fungus *Cordyceps sinensis* and the larval body of the host insect, which belongs to the Hepialidae family. Warm in nature with a sweet taste, it enters the lung and kidney meridians. It is effective in nourishing the lung and kidney, stopping bleeding, and transforming phlegm. It can be used to benefit those who are often sick and to treat diseases like pulmonary tuberculosis, chronic nephritis, and impotence. Cordyceps can nourish lung and kidney yang, and is highly effective in cases where yin deficiency leads to floating yang, manifesting as asthmatic breathing or coughing up blood. It has recently been popular as a tonic, but is contraindicated in cases with exterior symptoms or where there is lung heat causing bloody coughs.

Bajitian (Morindae Officinalis Radix)

Originated from the root of the *Morinda officinalis*, a plant in the Rubiaceae family, it is slightly warm with pungent and sweet flavors, and targets the kidney and liver meridians. It is known for its ability to strengthen kidney yang, fortify the sinews and bones, and dispel cold and dampness. It can be used to treat frequent urination, impotence due to kidney yang deficiency, rheumatic pain, and abdominal pain due to cold. Bajitian is suitable for treating deficiency-cold syndrome, but should be avoided by those with yin deficiency leading to excessive internal heat, dry mouth, and constipation.

Section 3
Commonly Used Famous Formulas for Nourishing the Body and Prolonging Life

What are the principles of formulating prescriptions for nourishing the body and prolonging life?

Formulas for nourishing the body and promoting longevity are often designed for the elderly and those with weakened constitutions, making supplementation the primary treatment method. The main principles for composing these formulas are as follows.

Principle 1: Integration of dynamic and static elements

These formulas often include tonic herbs, which tend to be rich and sticky, representing the "static" aspect as they nourish but do not move easily. To ensure these tonic effects reach the disease sites and are effectively dispersed, it is necessary to include herbs that invigorate qi and activate blood circulation, representing the "dynamic" aspect. This combination enhances both nourishment and circulation, resulting in a synergistic effect.

Principle 2: Combination of tonic and reducing herbs

Combining tonic and reducing herbs is a common formulation strategy. It balances nourishing and reducing actions to achieve harmony between yin and yang and balance qi and blood. A well-known kidney-yin tonic, Liuwei Dihuang Pills, exemplifies this principle with three tonic medicinals (Shanzhuyu, Shudihuang, Shanyao) and three purging herbs. In this formula, the "three tonic medicinals" refer to Shudihuang (Rehmanniae Radix Praeparata), Shanzhuyu (Corni Fructus) and Shanyao (Dioscoreae Rhizoma). Shudihuang (Rehmanniae Radix Praeparata) nourishes yin and replenishes the kidney, Shanzhuyu (Corni Fructus) nourishes the kidney and benefits the liver, while Shanyao (Dioscoreae Rhizoma) can simultaneously support the liver, spleen, and kidney. This balance prevents the cloying effects of tonics and facilitates absorption, harmonizing liver and kidney function. The "three purging medicinals" refer to Mudanpi (Moutan Cortex), Fuling (Poria), and Zexie (Alismatis Radix). These help to clear liver fire, drain dampness, and eliminate turbidity, preventing the overly rich and cloying nature of tonic medicinals from hindering the absorption of the medication. Together, these medicinals work in harmony to enhance the function of nourishing the liver and kidney.

Principle 3: Balancing heat and cold

Herbal properties are categorized into hot, cold, warm, and cool. It is crucial not to overly lean towards any extreme as too much cold can damage yang, while too much heat can harm yin. Formulations often pair hot and cold herbs to achieve a balanced effect, ensuring that the remedy is neither excessively cold nor overly drying. For instance, in Han Mao's famous formula for insomnia, Jiaotai Pills, the cold herb Huanglian (Coptidis Rhizoma) is paired with the warm herb Rougui (Cinnamomi Cortex), balancing each other to effectively treat heart and kidney disharmony.

Principle 4: Mutual enhancement and counteraction

The formulation of body-nourishing and life-prolonging prescriptions is based on differential diagnosis and takes a holistic approach. Each herb within a formula is selected not only for its primary effects but also for its ability to address secondary concerns, ensuring a structured, rigorous composition. Herbs that open and close, tonify and reduce, ascend and descend, and warm and cool are used together, complementing each other to enhance the formula's overall effectiveness.

What are the efficacies and applications of body-nourishing and life-prolonging prescriptions?

The primary ingredients in these formulas are tonic herbs, designed for treating deficiency patterns. The effects are threefold: enhancing the body's resistance and immune function; nourishing deficiency and regulating physiological functions; and providing anti-aging benefits and extending life. These formulas are suitable for conditions such as congenital insufficiency, physical weakness post-illness or postpartum, weakness in the elderly, and as adjuvent theray for cancer. They are also used for preventive health care and life extension.

What are the common dosage forms of body-nourishing and life-prolonging prescriptions?

Ancient wisdom thinks different forms for different purposes: decoctions for major illnesses, powders for urgent conditions, and pills for chronic conditions. Common forms include decoction, powder, pill, paste, and pellet. In addition, medicinal wine, meal and tea are also frequently used.

Decoction: Herbal ingredients are soaked and boiled to create a liquid form, taken orally. They are characterized by fast absorption and rapid action.

Powder: Herbs are ground into a fine powder, easy to produce, and stable, suitable for internal and external use.

Pill: Including honey pills, water pills, paste pills, and concentrated pills, these are made by mixing powdered herbs with binders like honey, water, flour or rice paste, or medicinal juice. Pills are small, easy to store, have long-lasting potency, and are absorbed slowly.

Paste: Also known as gaozi or gaofang, are made by condensing decoctions and adding excipients. It is popular in Jiangnan region of China for winter supplementation due to their smooth, pleasant texture and dual function in nourishment and treatment.

Pellet: Mainly composed of refined or precious medicinal ingredients, is referred to as "dan (pellet)" instead of "wan (pill)" formulation. Some powdered formulations with small dosage but significant effects are also called "dan". Certain surgical dan formulations contain minerals such as mercury and sulfur. They are prepared by heating and sublimation, and possess the characteristics of small dosage, strong effect, and mineral content. Examples include Hongsheng Pellet and Baijiang Pellet. Additionally, certain expensive or uniquely efficacious medicinal formulations are colloquially referred to as "dan", such as Zhibao Pellet and Zixue Pellet. Therefore, dan formulation does not refer to a fixed type of formulation.

Medicinal wine: Herbs are infused in alcohol or rice wine, after the active components are dissovled in the liquid, then it is filtered for, internal or external use. Alcohol is a good semi-polar organic solvent, and various active ingredients in Chinese medicinals easily dissolve in it. By harnessing the power of alcohol, the medicinal efficacy of medicinals can be fully exerted, leading to improved therapeutic effects. Famous medicinal wines that have been passed down through generations include Yujiaotang, while emerging ones include Guishoujiu and Jingjiu. According to TCM theory, chronic deficiency-based diseases will eventually lead to weakened vital energy and stagnant meridians. Medicinal wines are formulated to nourish the blood, tonify qi, nourish yin, and warm yang. Moreover, alcohol itself has the effects of dispersing and promoting circulation. Therefore, medicinal wines can be widely used in the prevention and treatment of various chronic deficiency-based diseases, as well as have anti-aging and longevity-promoting benefits.

Medicated diet, as a combination of medicine and food, refers to a type of dietary therapy that involves cooking and processing medicinal ingredients. It is a product of the integration of traditional Chinese medical knowledge and culinary experience. Medicated diet incorporates medicine into food by using medicinal substances as ingredients and giving medicinal properties to the food. By leveraging the power of food and assisting the efficacy of medicine, medicated diet serves as a special type of diet that combines medicinal effects with culinary delights. It not only provides nutritional value but also helps prevent and treat diseases, promote health, and prolong life.

Medicinal tea, also known as herbal tea, refers to a preparation in which Chinese herbal medicine is combined with tea leaves, or Chinese herbal medicine (single or compound) or crude powder is brewed or boiled like tea for consumption. Medicinal tea is a traditional dosage form in China, developed under the guidance of TCM theories, principles, formulas, and pharmacology. It is formulated according to syndrome differentiation or a combination of syndrome differentiation and disease identification, for the purpose of preventing and treating diseases, post-disease recovery, or health preservation. Medicinal tea has the characteristics of convenient preparation, strong targeting, and high flexibility, making it suitable for disease treatment and health restoration. It retains the flexibility and remarkable therapeutic effects of traditional Chinese herbal decoctions based on syndrome differentiation, while overcoming the drawbacks of complex decoction processes and inconvenience in carrying. It aligns with the development trend of a fast-paced modern lifestyle.

What is the classification of body-nourishing and life-prolonging formulas?

Based on their primary actions, these formulas can be categorized into types, such as nourish the heart, liver, spleen, lung, kidney, and all five organs. Additionally, there are categories for beauty and complexion enhancement and brain and intellect fortification. Each category targets specific types of deficiency and imbalance.

Exalted Formulas for Nurturing the Heart

Shenxian Baojing Yanzhu Erfuling Formula (from *Taiping Holy Beneficence Prescription*)

Composition: Fuling (Poria), Songzhi (pine resin), Zhongrufen (stalactite powder), Baifengmi (white honey).

Function: Nourishes the heart and kidney, enhances vitality and spirit.

Indications: Insufficiency of the heart and kidney, restlessness, insomnia, forgetfulness, and lack of strength.

Sibu Pills (from *Shengji General Record*)

Composition: Baiziren (Platycladi Semen), Heshouwu (Polygoni Multiflori Radix), Roucongrong (Cistanches Herba), Niuxi (Achyranthis Bidentatae Radix).

Function: Tonifies the kidney, nourishes the heart, and calms the spirit.

Indications: Kidney deficiency, insufficient heart and mental energy, insomnia, forgetfulness, and weakness in the lumbar region and knees.

Dingzhi Buxin Decoction (from *A Supplement to Recipes Worth A Thousand Gold*)

Composition: Yuanzhi (Polygalae Radix), Changpu (Acori Tatarinowii Rhizoma), Renshen (Ginseng Radix et Rhizoma), Fuling (Poria).

Function: Augments heart qi.

Indications: Deficiency of heart qi, heart pain, and panic.

Yangxin Yanling Yishou Pills (from *Medical Formulary Selected by Empress Dowager Cixi*)

Composition: Fushen (Poria with hostwood), Danggui (Angelicae Sinensis

Radix), Jiubaishao (Paeoniae Radix Alba, prepared with wine), Mudanpi (Moutan Cortex), Dihuang (Rehmanniae Radix), Chaozhiqiao (Aurantii Fructus, dry-fried), Suanzaoren (Ziziphi Spinosae Semen), Danshen (Salviae Miltiorrhizae Radix et Rhizoma), Baiziren (Platycladi Semen), Chuanxiong (Chuanxiong Rhizoma), Chaobaizhu (Atractylodis Macrocephalae Rhizoma, dry-fried), Chenpi (Citri Reticulatae Pericarpium), Jiuhuangqin (Scutellariae Radix, prepared with wine), Zhizi (Gardeniae Fructus).

Function: Nurtures the heart, calms the spirit, enriches the blood, and softens the liver.

Indications: Liver fire and depressed heat, loss of nourishment in the heart and mind, physical frailty, timidness, difficulty in sleeping, dry throat, and heat in the soles of the feet.

Exalted Formulas for Nurturing the Liver

Mingmu Yishen Pills (from *Teachings of [Zhu] Danxi*)

Composition: Gouqizi (Lycii Fructus), Danggui (Angelicae Sinensis Radix), Shengdihuang (Rehmanniae Radix), Fushen (Poria with hostwood), Tusizi (Cuscutae Semen), Zhimu (Anemarrhenae Rhizoma), Huangbo (Phellodendri Chinensis Cortex), Shanyao (Dioscoreae Rhizoma), Bajitian (Morindae Officinalis Radix), Wuweizi (Schisandrae Chinensis Fructus), Tiandong (Asparagi Radix), Renshen (Ginseng Radix et Rhizoma), Juhua (Chrysanthemi Flos).

Function: Nourishes yin, fortifies the kidney, and clears and nurtures the liver and eyes.

Indications: Deficiency of liver and kidney, excessive kidney fire, insufficient qi and yin, dizziness, and blurred vision.

Mingmu Yanling Paste (from *Selected Prescriptions of Empress Dowager Cixi*)

Composition: Sangye (Mori Folium), Juhua (Chrysanthemi Flos).
Function: Softens the liver and brightens the eyes.
Indications: Predominant liver fire, dizziness, and blurred vision.

Shenxian Zhuyan Yannian Formula (from *Universal Relief Prescriptions*)

Composition: Zhishi (Aurantii Immaturus Fructus), Shudihuang (Rehmanniae

Radix Praeparata), Juhua (Chrysanthemi Flos), Tiandong (Asparagi Radix).

Function: Nourishes the liver and kidneys, clarifies vision.

Indications: Insufficiency of liver and kidney, blurred vision, feeling of fullness below the heart.

Qiju Dihuang Pills (from *Medical Ranks*)

Composition: Gouqizi (Lycii Fructus), Juhua (Chrysanthemi Flos), Shudihuang (Rehmanniae Radix Praeparata), Shanzhuyu (Corni Fructus), Shanyao (Dioscoreae Rhizoma), Fuling (Poria), Zexie (Alismatis Radix), Mudanpi (Moutan Cortex).

Function: Strengthens the kidney, nurtures the liver, and brightens the eyes.

Indications: Deficiency of liver and kidney, dizziness, blurred vision, excessive thirst.

Exalted Formulas for Nurturing the Spleen

Shouzhong Pills (from *Shengji General Record*)

Composition: Shengdihuang (Rehmanniae Radix), Renshen (Ginseng Radix et Rhizoma), Baizhu (Atractylodis Macrocephalae Rhizoma), Juhua (Chrysanthemi Flos), Shanyao (Dioscoreae Rhizoma), Gouqizi (Lycii Fructus), Fuling (Poria), Maidong (Ophiopogonis Radix).

Function: Augments qi, strengthens the spleen, benefits the kidney, and nourishes the liver.

Indications: Deficiency of acquired constitution, loss of prenatal nourishment, dizziness, discomfort in the loins and ribs, emaciation.

Jianpi Decoction (from *A Supplement to Recipes Worth A Thousand Gold*)

Composition: Shengdihuang (Rehmanniae Radix), Huangqi (Astragali Radix), Shaoyao (Paeoniae Radix), Gancao (Glycyrrhizae Radix et Rhizoma), Shengjiang (fresh ginger), Baimi (white honey).

Function: Nourishes yin blood and strengthens the spleen and stomach.

Indications: Disharmony of qi and blood, heaviness as if weighted by stone, desire to eat followed by vomiting, soreness in limbs.

Fuyuan Hezhong Paste (from *Selected Prescriptions of Empress Dowager Cixi*)

Composition: Dangshen (Codonopsis Radix), Baizhu (Atractylodis

Macrocephalae Rhizoma), Fuling (Poria), Dangguishen (Angelicae Sinensis Radix, the body part), Duzhong (Eucommiae Cortex), Huangqi (Astragali Radix), Chaoguya (Setariae Fructus Germinatus, dry-fired), Jineijin (Galli Gigeriae Endothelium Corneum), Sharen (Amomi Fructus), Peilan (Eupatorii Herba), Xiangfu (Cyperi Rhizoma), Shengjiang (fresh ginger), Jiangbanxia (Pinelliae Rhizoma Praeparatum cum Zingibere et Alumine), Dazao (Jujubae Fructus).

Function: Supports the primal qi and harmonizes the middle.

Indications: Chronic spleen deficiency with reduced appetite, chest tightness, dry retching, feeling of fullness after eating, and indigestion.

Muxiang Renshen Powder (from *New Book on Elderly Care for Parents' Longevity*)

Composition: Muxiang (Aucklandiae Radix), Renshen (Ginseng Radix et Rhizoma), Baizhu (Atractylodis Macrocephalae Rhizoma), Dingxiang (Caryophylli Flos), Zhigancao (Glycyrrhizae Radix et Rhizoma Praeparata cum Melle), Houpo (Magnoliae Officinalis Cortex), Ganjiang (Zingiberis Rhizoma), Chenpi (Citri Reticulatae Pericarpium), Fuling (Poria), Roudoukou (Myristicae Semen), Pipaye (Eriobotryae Folium), Huoxiangye (Pogostemonis Folium).

Function: Warms the middle and regulates qi.

Indications: The elderly with spleen and stomach deficiency and cold, epigastric and abdominal distending pain, reverse flow of phlegm and vomiting, disorderly stools.

Exalted Formulas for Nurturing the Lung

Qiongyu Paste (from *Teachings of [Zhu] Danxi*)

Composition: Renshen (Ginseng Radix et Rhizoma), Fuling (Poria), Shengdihuang (Rehmanniae Radix), Baimi (white honey).

Function: Benefits qi and yin, nourishes the heart and lung.

Indication: Debilitating cough, shortness of breath, and lack of strength.

Bufei Powder (from *A Supplement to Recipes Worth A Thousand Gold*)

Composition: Baishiying (Quartz Album), Wuweizi (Schisandrae Chinensis Fructus), Guixin (Cinnamomi Cortex), Dazao (Jujubae Fructus), Maidong (Ophiopogonis Radix), Kuandonghua (Farfarae Flos), Sangbaipi (Mori Cortex),

Ganjiang (Zingiberis Rhizoma), Gancao (Glycyrrhizae Radix et Rhizoma).

Function: Warms the heart and kidney, and augments lung qi.

Indications: Insufficiency of lung qi, chest pain radiating to the back, loss of voice due to qi ascent.

Exalted Formulas for Nurturing the Kidney

Tusizi Pills (from *Formulas to Aid the Living*)

Composition: Tusizi (Cuscutae Semen), Duzhong (Eucommiae Cortex), Shudihuang (Rehmanniae Radix Praeparata), Lurong (Cervi Cornu Pantotrichum), Roucongrong (Cistanches Herba), Cheqianzi (Plantaginis Semen), Guixin (Cinnamomi Cortex), Niuxi (Achyranthis Bidentatae Radix), Fuzi (Aconiti Lateralis Radix Praeparata).

Function: Warms and supplements kidney yang.

Indications: Cold and soreness in the loins and knees, cold limbs, impotence, and female infertility due to cold uterus.

Da Buyin Pills (from *Teachings of [Zhu] Danxi*)

Composition: Chaohuangbo (Phellodendri Chinensis Cortex, dry-fried), Chaozhimu (Anemarrhenae Rhizoma, dry-fried), Shudihuang (Rehmanniae Radix Praeparata), Guijia (Testudinis Carapax et Plastrum).

Function: Nourishes yin and reduces fire.

Indications: Yin deficiency with hyperactive fire, tidal fever, night sweating, weakness, and debilitation.

Erzhi Pills (from *Universal Relief Prescriptions*)

Composition: Nvzhenzi (Ligustri Lucidi Fructus), Mohanlian (Ecliptae Herba).

Function: Nourishes yin and enriches blood.

Indications: Yin deficiency, insufficient liver and kidney, dizziness, insomnia, soreness in the loins and knees, and premature greying of hair.

Yanshou Pills (from *Shi Bu Zhai Medical Book*)

Composition: Heshouwu (Polygoni Multiflori Radix), Xixiancao (Siegesbeckiae Herba), Tusizi (Cuscutae Semen), Duzhong (Eucommiae Cortex), Niuxi (Achyranthis Bidentatae Radix), Nvzhenzi (Ligustri Lucidi

Fructus), Sangye (Mori Folium), Rendongteng (Lonicerae Japonicae Caulis), Shengdihuang (Rehmanniae Radix), Sangshen paste (mulberry paste), Heizhima paste (black sesame paste), Jinyingzi paste (roselle paste), Mohanlian paste (drynaria paste).

Function: Nourishes the kidney and liver, strengthens sinews and bones, and dispels wind.

Indications: Deficiency of liver and kidney, decline of yin and blood, dizziness, lumbar pain, premature greying of hair, and premature aging.

Yishou Yangzhen Paste (from *Treasure Mirror of Eastern Medicine*)

Composition: Shengdihuang (Rehmanniae Radix), Renshen (Ginseng Radix et Rhizoma), Fuling (Poria), Tiandong (Asparagi Radix), Maidong (Ophiopogonis Radix), Digupi (Lycii Cortex), Mi (Mel).

Function: Augments qi, nourishes yin, fills essence, and replenishes marrow.

Indications: General debility, paralysis, consumptive diseases, insufficient vitality of the five viscera, and lack of mental vigor.

Exalted Formulas for Nurturing the Five Zang Organs

Yangshou Pellet (from *Imperial Pharmacy Prescriptions*)

Composition: Yuanzhi (Polygalae Radix), Changpu (Acori Tatarinowii Rhizoma), Bajitian (Morindae Officinalis Radix), Baizhu (Atractylodis Macrocephalae Rhizoma), Fuling (Poria), Digupi (Lycii Cortex), Xuduan (Dipsaci Radix), Gouqizi (Lycii Fructus), Juhua (Chrysanthemi Flos), Xixin (Asari Radix et Rhizoma), Dihuang (Rehmanniae Radix), Cheqianzi (Plantaginis Semen), Heshouwu (Polygoni Multiflori Radix), Niuxi (Achyranthis Bidentatae Radix), Roucongrong (Cistanches Herba), Tusizi (Cuscutae Semen), Fupenzi (Rubi Fructus).

Function: Supplements and nourishes the five zang viscera.

Indications: Deficiency and damage to the five zang viscera, numbness and pain, premature greying of hair, and weakness of sinews and bones.

Banlong Erzhi Baibu Pills (from *Complete Book of Jingyue*)

Composition: Lujiao (Cervi Cornu), Huangjing (Polygonati Rhizoma), Gouqizi (Lycii Fructus), Shudihuang (Rehmanniae Radix Praeparata), Tusizi (Cuscutae Semen), Jinyingzi (Rosae Laevigatae Fructus), Tiandong (Asparagi

Radix), Maidong (Ophiopogonis Radix), Niuxi (Achyranthis Bidentatae Radix), Chushizi (Broussonetiae Fructus), Longyanrou (Longan Arillus), Lujiaoshuang (Cervi Cornu Degelatinatum), Renshen (Ginseng Radix et Rhizoma), Huangqi (Astragali Radix), Qianshi (Euryales Semen), Fuling (Poria), Shanyao (Dioscoreae Rhizoma), Shanzhuyu (Corni Fructus), Shengdihuang (Rehmanniae Radix), Zhimu (Anemarrhenae Rhizoma), Wuweizi (Schisandrae Chinensis Fructus).

Function: Consolidates the foundation and protects the origin, regulates the five zang organs.

Indications: Deficiency and damage to the five zang viscera, emaciation with fever of the bones, or male infertility.

Exalted Formulas for Beauty and Facial Care

Qibai Powder (from *Eternal Categories Seal Formulas*)

Composition: Bailian (Ampelopsis Radix), Baizhu (Atractylodis Macrocephalae Rhizoma), Baiqianniu (Pharbitidis Semen, white), Baifuzi (Typhonii Rhizoma), Baizhi (Angelicae Dahuricae Radix), Baishao (Paeoniae Radix Alba), Baijiangcan (Bombyx Batryticatus).

Usage: Remove the outer layers from all herbs except the Baijiangcan. Grind all the medicinals into a powder, store in a bottle, and use to wash the face in the morning and evening.

Function: Whitens and refines the skin.

Qibao Meiran Pills (from *Compendium of Materia Medica* cited from *Ji Shan Tang Formulas*)

Composition: Heshouwu (Polygoni Multiflori Radix), Fuling (Poria), Niuxi (Achyranthis Bidentatae Radix), Danggui (Angelicae Sinensis Radix), Gouqizi (Lycii Fructus), Tusizi (Cuscutae Semen), Buguzhi (Psoraleae Fructus).

Usage: Form into pills with honey, taken with salt broth or alcohol.

Function: Treats liver and kidneydeficiency, and premature greying of hair.

Exalted Formulas for Enhancing Brain Function and Wisdom

Qisheng Pills (from *Shengji General Record*)

Composition: Fuling (Poria), Renshen (Ginseng Radix et Rhizoma), Tiandong

(Asparagi Radix), Yuanzhi (Polygalae Radix), Changpu (Acori Tatarinowii Rhizoma), Digupi (Lycii Cortex), Rougui (Cinnamomi Cortex).

Function: Enhances mental acuity and wisdom.

Indications: Heart deficiency causing forgetfulness.

Yangming Kaixin Yizhi Formula (from *Essential Recipes for Emergent Use Worth A Thousand Gold*)

Composition: Gandihuang (Rehmanniae Radix), Renshen (Ginseng Radix et Rhizoma), Fuling (Poria), Roucongrong (Cistanches Herba), Yuanzhi (Polygalae Radix), Tusizi (Cuscutae Semen), Shechuangzi (Cnidii Fructus).

Function: Supplements the kidney, nourishes the heart, and enhances intelligence.

Indications: Deficiency of heart and kidney, essence and blood insufficiency, forgetfulness, and insomnia.

What should be considered when using formulas for health promotion and longevity?

While medications for health promotion and longevity have numerous benefits, it is imperative to adhere to the principles and contraindications of tonification. The esteemed Qing Dynasty doctor Cheng Guopeng once elucidated: "The purpose of tonification is profound indeed! However, errors occur when tonification is necessary but omitted, when it is unnecessarily administered, and when it is applied without distinguishing between qi and blood, identifying cold or heat syndromes, differentiating between opening and closing actions, assessing urgency, recognizing the specific organs involved, understanding the fundamental issues, or thoroughly pursuing the appropriate modulating strategies. These are critical aspects that must be discussed" (*Insights into Medicine*). In practice, tonification should be tailored to individual factors such as age, gender, occupation, living environment, season, and constitutional characteristics. TCM posits that tonic prescriptions for deficient conditions should follow six principles: treatment based on differential diagnosis (tailoring medications to the constitution and adapting to the three causative factors), avoiding indiscriminate tonification, preventing excessive bias in tonification, reducing excess conditions appropriately, ensuring that purgation does not harm the vital essence, and employing a gradual approach in medication use.

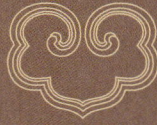

Chapter 7

Acupuncture and Moxibustion for

Health Preservation

Section 1
Overview of Acupuncture and Moxibustion for Health Preservation

What is acupuncture and moxibustion for health preservation?

Acupuncture for health preservation involves the use of acupuncture and moxibustion techniques to enhance health and prevent or treat diseases. "Acupuncture" refers to the method of needling. This therapeutic approach is based on the theory of organs and meridians, incorporating the Four Diagnoses and Eight Principles theory, along with a system of disease identification and differential diagnosis. It involves formulating a precise prescription of acupuncture points and applying techniques accordingly to unblock meridians, regulate qi and blood, and restore a relative balance between yin and yang, thereby achieving both preventative and curative effects. Common acupuncture therapies include filiform needle therapy, fire needle therapy, and electro-acupuncture. "Moxibustion" utilizes mugwort wool or other medicinal substances burnt at specific acupoints on the body. The heat from the moxa, along with the properties of the medicinal substances, is transmitted through the meridians, warming the meridians, supplementing the vital energy, regulating qi and blood, and warming the uterus to dispel cold, thus serving as another distinctive TCM treatment method for disease prevention and treatment.

What are the characteristics of acupuncture and moxibustion for health preservation?

First, it has a long history and rich practical experience. Second, it has definitive therapeutic effects and simple manipulation, which make acupuncture and moxibustion widely acceptable. Third, it can ben combined with other health care methods, thus enhancing the effects, such as qigong, massage, dietary therapy, and Chinese medicinals.

Section 2
Machanism of Acupuncture and Moxibustion for Health Preservation

What is the theoretical basis of acupuncture and moxibustion for health preservation?

Acupuncture and moxibustion for health preservation is founded on meridian theory. The meridian system comprizes channels and collaterals, including the twelve regular meridians, eight extraordinary meridians, fifteen subdivisions, etc. They form an intricate network that facilitates the connection between internal organs and the body, ensuring the smooth flow of qi and blood and nurturing the whole body. Acupuncture and moxibustion target specific acupoints or meridian pathways to stimulate and balance the body's metabolic processes, thereby strengthening the body and extending life.

What are the effects of acupuncture and moxibustion?

First, supporting the body's vitality and expelling pathogens, and enhancing the immune function. Acupuncture has a beneficial bidirectional regulatory effect; it can tonify deficiency to support the body's vitality and reduce excess to expel pathogens. Although the methods of acupuncture for health maintenance and treating diseases are fundamentally similar, their focuses differ. Acupuncture for disease treatment focuses on correcting imbalances of yin and yang, and qi and blood in the body, while acupuncture for health maintenance aims at strengthening the body and enhancing its metabolic capacity, with the goal of health preservation and longevity. Due to these different focuses, there are some differences in point selection and needling techniques. For health maintenance, the intensity of stimulation should be moderate, with a limited number of acupuncture points, primarily those with strengthening effects. Moxibustion for health maintenance is a unique Chinese method for health preservation, which can be used not only for strengthening and maintaining health but also for the rehabilitation of those with chronic illnesses and physical weakness. The so-called health maintenance moxibustion involves applying moxibustion on certain specific points to achieve the purpose of harmonizing qi and blood, regulating the meridians, nourishing the organs, and prolonging life. As stated in *Introduction to Medicine*: "Where medicine does not reach, and needles do not penetrate, so moxibustion is necessary." It indicates that moxibustion can sometimes achieve what acupuncture and medicine cannot. The health maintenance effects of moxibustion were clearly recorded in the *Bianque Xinshu*: "When a person is free from illness, frequently apply moxibustion to Guānyuán (CV4), Qìhǎi (CV6), Mìngmén (GV4), and Zhōngwǎn (CV12) points...Even if it does not grant eternal life, it can ensure a lifespan of over a hundred years."

Second, balancing yin and yang, and adjusting organ functions. The balance of yin and yang is the physiological state of a healthy person, and the goal of acupuncture and moxibustion for health preservation is to adjust and maintain this state. *Miraculous Pivot–Genjie* states: "The key to using needles lies in knowing how to regulate yin and yang. When yin and yang are regulated, vitality is bright, and the form and qi are harmonized, allowing the spirit to reside within." This illustrates that acupuncture and moxibustionhasthe function of balancing yin and yang and adjusting organ functions. This is accomplished through the yin-yang properties of the meridians, point combinations, and acupuncture and moxibustion techniques.

Third, unblocking the meridians and harmonizing qi and blood. Qi and blood are the material foundation of human life activities, relying on the transmission through the meridians throughout the body, playing roles such as propulsion, warming, transformation, consolidation, defense, and nutrition. Only when the meridians are unblocked and qi and blood are harmonized can the organ functions operate normally, allowing physical and mental well-being. Through certain acupuncture techniques and appropriate stimulation at acupuncture points, the blocked meridians can be unblocked, allowing them to perform their normal physiological functions, thereby achieving the goal of prolonging life.

Section 3
Applications of Acupuncture and Moxibustion for Health Preservation

What are the indications for acupuncture therapy?

Acupuncture is effective for various conditions, including neurological disorders such as idopathic facial paralysis, sequelae of cerebrovascular accidents, motor neuron disease, and spinal cord injuries; various neuralgias like postherpetic neuralgia, numbness and pain caused by diabetic peripheral neuropathy, trigeminal neuralgia, etc.; musculoskeletal disorders such as cervical spondylosis, lumbar spondylosis, osteoarthritis, frozen shoulder, and acute sprains; internal medicine diseases such as rheumatoid arthritis, ankylosing spondylitis, chronic gastroenteritis, and irritable bowel syndrome; gynecological disorders such as menstrual disorders, and premature ovarian failure; urinary system diseases such as urinary retention, and urinary incontinence; ENT (ear, nose, and throat) diseases such as allergic rhinitis, and optic atrophy. It is also beneficial for mild anxiety, sleep disorders, subhealth states, and cosmetic purposes such as weight loss and skin beautification.

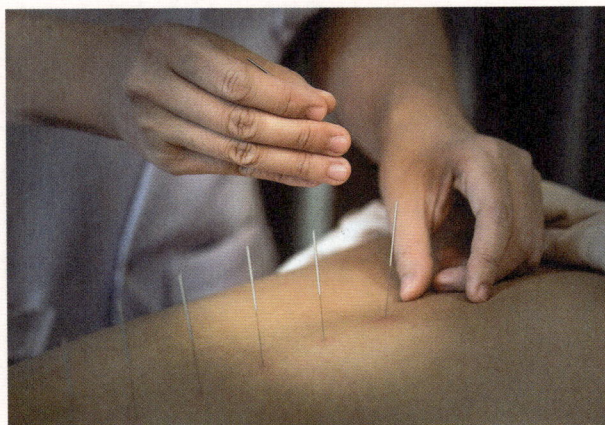

Acupuncture manipulation

What are the contraindications and precautions for acupuncture therapy?

Contraindications: Intoxication, unstable emotional states, or psychosis; infectious skin diseases or injuries.

Precautions: Do not undergoing therapy on an empty or overly full stomach; after treatment, keep warm and avoid eating cold and uncooked foods.

What are the indications for moxibustion therapy?

Moxibustion therapy can be applied to the following conditions: limited joint movement and muscle stiffness caused by cold-induced blood stasis and blockage of the meridians; dysmenorrhea and menstrual irregularities in women caused by cold congealing the meridians; abdominal pain, diarrhea, bloating, and constipation caused by middle jiao deficiency and cold; impotence, nocturnal emission, insomnia with excessive dreaming, and frequent nighttime urination caused by kidney yang deficiency; chronic, non-healing ulcers; optic nerve atrophy; and postherpetic neuralgia.

What are the indications and contraindications for moxibustion?

Contraindications: Moxibustion should not be applied to the lumbar and abdominal areas of pregnant women; individuals who are extremely fatigued, overly hungry or full, emotionally unstable, or intoxicated; those allergic to mugwort or prone to skin allergies; and those with excess heat syndromes or yin deficiency with fever.

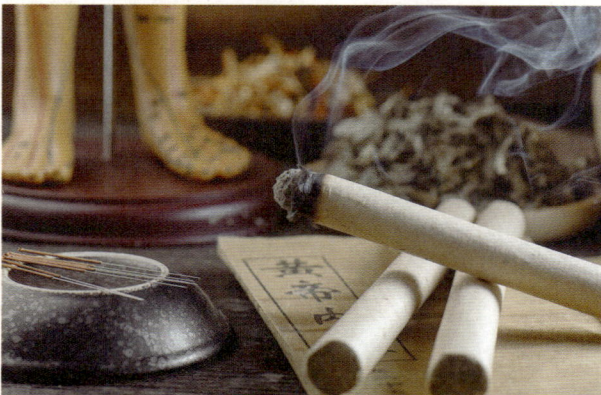

Moxibustion

Precautions: After moxibustion, avoid exposure to wind and cold; it is not advisable to perform moxibustion immediately after meals—waiting one hour after eating is recommended; avoid drinking cold water or consuming raw and cold foods immediately after moxibustion; a temporary feeling of fatigue may occur after moxibustion, which is a normal phenomenon and can be alleviated with a short rest.

Common acupoints for health maintenance in acupuncture and moxibustion

Common acupoints: Hégǔ (LI4), Zúsānlǐ (ST36), Fēngmén (BL12), Gāohuāng (BL43), Guānyuán (CV4), Qìhǎi (CV6), Shénquè (CV8), Dàzhuī (GV14), Yǒngquán (KI1).

Hégǔ (LI4)

Location: On the dorsum of the hand, between the 1st and 2nd metacarpal bones, approximately at the midpoint of the radial side of the 2nd metacarpal bone.

Efficacy: Resustates the mind and opens the orifices, dispels wind and clears heat, alleviates pain, and dredges meridians.

Manipulation: Perpendicular inserts 0.5–1 cun. Moxibustion is applicable.

Indications: Disorders of the head and face, heat boils, anhidrosis, spontaneous sweating, night sweating, amenorrhea, delayed labor, coma, and epilepsy.

Combination: Tonifies Hégǔ (LI4) and reduces Fùliū (KI7) to induce sweating; reduces Hégǔ (LI4) and tonifies Fùliū (KI7) to stop sweating.

Combines with Fēngchí (GB20), Dàzhuī (GV14), and Qūchí (LI11) to

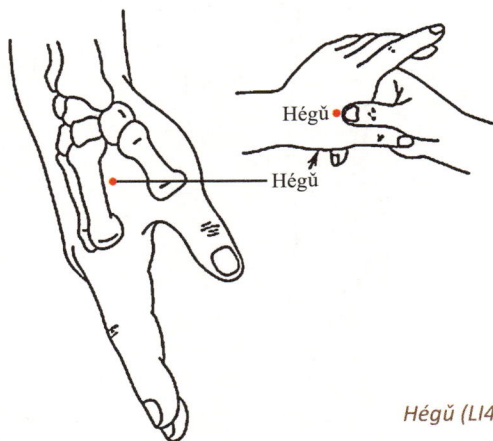

Hégǔ (LI4)

treat external febrile diseases.

Combines with Xiàguān (ST7) and Jiáchē (ST6) to treat toothache.

Combines with Qūchí (LI11), Fēngshì (GB31) and Géshù (BL17) to treat systemic urticaria.

Zúsānlǐ (ST36)

Location: On the lateral side of the lower leg, 3 cun below Dúbí (ST35), on the line connecting Dúbí (ST35) and Jiěxī (ST41).

Efficacy: Strengthens the spleen and stomach, regulates qi and blood, and supports the body's vital energy.

Manipulation: Perpendicular inserts 1–2 cun. Moxibustion is applicable.

Indications: Gastric pain, abdominal distention, vomiting, diarrhea, constipation, hypertension, neurasthenia, weakness and paralysis of the lower limbs.

Combination: Combines with Nèiguān (PC6) and Zhōngwǎn (CV12) to treat gastric pain.

Combines with Qūchí (LI11) and Tàichōng (LR3) to treat hypertension.

Combines with Qūchí (LI11) to treat urticaria.

Combines with Shuǐgōu (GV26), Nèiguān (PC6), and Bǎihuì (GV20) to treat shock.

Regular moxibustion on Zúsānlǐ (ST36) can not only regulate the digestive system and prevent gastrointestinal diseases but also has the effects of strengthening the body and prolonging life.

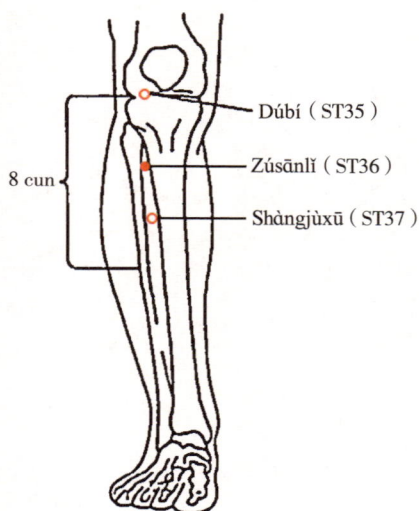

8 cun
Dúbí (ST35)
Zúsānlǐ (ST36)
Shàngjùxū (ST37)

Zúsānlǐ (ST36)

Fēngmén (BL12)

Location: On the back, 1.5 cun lateral to the posterior median line, under the spinous process of the 2nd thoracic vertebra.

Efficacy: Dispels wind and releases the exterior, clears heat and ventilatets the lung.

Manipulation: Perpendicularly inserts 0.5–1 cun. Moxibustion is applicable.

Indications: Common cold, cough, headache, fever, urticaria, stiff neck, back pain.

Combination: Combines with Dàzhuī (GV14), Fèishù (BL13) and Kǒngzuì (LU6) to treat external febrile cough.

Combines with Fēngchí (GB20) and Xuèhǎi (SP10) to treat urticaria.

Combines with Fēngchí (GB20) and Lièquē (LU7) to treat common cold headache.

Gāohuāng (BL43)

Location: On the back, 3 cun lateral to the posterior median line, under the spinous process of the 4th thoracic vertebra.

Efficacy: Regulates lung qi and replenishes deficiency.

Manipulation: Obliquely inserts 0.5–0.8 cun. Moxibustion is applicable.

Indications: Pulmonary tuberculosis, cough and asthma, hemoptysis, night sweating, spleen and stomach deficiency, and scapular pain.

Combination: Combines with Guānyuán (CV4) and Zúsānlǐ (ST36) with moxibustion to treat chronic weakness and emaciation.

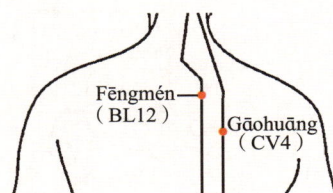

Fēngmén (BL12) and Gāohuāng (BL43)

Guānyuán (CV4)

Location: On the lower abdomen, 4 cun below the umbilicus, on the anterior midline.

Efficacy: Warms the kidney and consolidates essence, tonifies qi and restores yang, clears heat and resolves dampness.

Manipulation: Perpendicularly inserts 1–2 cun. Contraindicated in pregnancy.

Indications: Abdominal pain, irregular menstruation, leukorrhea, female infertility, seminal emission, hernia, frequent urination.

Combination: Combines with Dàimài (GB26) and Sānyīnjiāo (SP6) to treat excessive leukorrhea.

Combines with Sānyīnjiāo (SP6) and Yīnlíngquán (SP9) to treat seminal emission.

Qìhǎi (CV6)

Location: On the lower abdomen, 1.5 cun below the umbilicus, on the anterior midline.

Efficacy: Raises and supplements yang qi, tonifies deficiency and consolidates the origin.

Manipulation: Perpendicularly inserts 1–2 cun.

Indications: Lower abdominal pain, irregular menstruation, seminal emission, stroke of collapse type, leukorrhea, menorrhagia and metrostaxis, female infertility, hernia, and rectal prolapse.

Combination: Combines with Zhōngjí (CV3), Shènshù (BL23), Sānyīnjiāo (SP6) and Xíngjiān (LR2) to treat red and white leukorrhea.

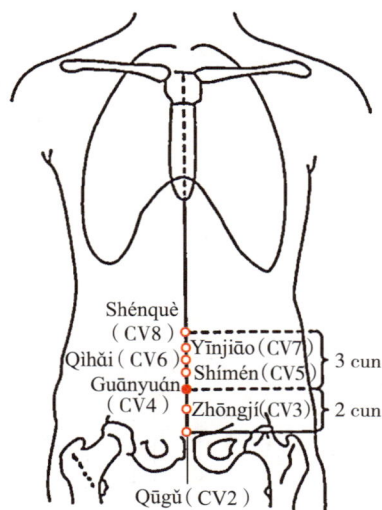

Guānyuán (CV4), Qìhǎi (CV6) and Shénquè (CV8)

Combines with Guīlái (ST29) to treat enuresis.

Shénquè (CV8)

Location: In the center of the umbilicus.

Efficacy: Restores yang and rescues from collapse, strengthens the spleen and stomach.

Manipulation: Needle insertion is prohibited. Moxibustion for 5–15 minutes.

Indications: Stroke of collapse type, abdominal gurgling, rectal prolapse, persistent diarrhea, dysentery, and abdominal pain.

Combination: Combines with Zúsānlǐ (ST36) to treat borborygmus and abdominal pain

Combines with Changqiang (GV1) and Qìhǎi (CV6) to treat rectal prolapse.

Combines with Qìhǎi (CV6) and Yīnlíngquán (SP9) to treat diarrhea.

Combines with Guānyuán (CV4) to treat stroke of collapse type.

Cupping on Shénquè (CV8) combines with puncturing Tiānshū (ST25) and Zúsānlǐ (ST36) to treat diarrhea and vomiting.

Dàzhuī (GV14)

Location: On the posterior median line, in the depression below the spinous process of the 7th cervical vertebra.

Efficacy: Releases the exterior and clears heat, resustates the mind and clears the brain.

Manipulation: Inserts upward obliquely 0.5–1 cun.

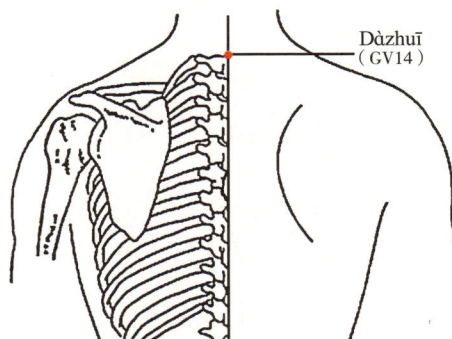

Dàzhuī
(GV14)

Dàzhuī (GV14)

Indications: Stiff neck and pain, chest

and rib pain, shoulder and back pain, headache, fever, malaria, epilepsy, cough, and asthma.

Combination: Combines with Qūchí (LI11) and Hégǔ (LI4) to treat influenza.

Combines with Fēnglóng (ST40) to treat cough.

Combines with Zúsānlǐ (ST36) and Qūchí (LI11) to treat leukopenia.

Yǒngquán (KI1)

Location: On the sole of the foot, in the depression formed when the foot is in plantar flexion.

Efficacy: Clears heat, opens the orifices, and calms the mind.

Manipulation: Perpendicularly inserts 0.5–1 cun.

Indications: Headache, dizziness, coma due to stroke, shock, pediatric convulsions, dysuria, constipation, hot sensation and pain in the sole.

Combination: Combines with Guānyuán (CV4) and Fēnglóng (ST40) to treat consumptive cough.

Combines with Shuǐgōu (GV26) to treat pediatric convulsions.

Combines with Zúsānlǐ (ST36) to treat toxic shock.

Combines with Kūnlún (BL60) to treat constipation.

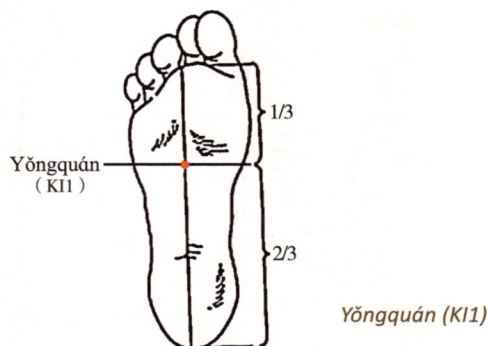

Yǒngquán (KI1)

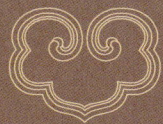

Chapter 8

Other Non-medication Therapy

for Health Preservation

Section 1
Overview of Non-medication Therapy for Health Preservation

What are the advantages of TCM non-medication therapy?

TCM non-medication therapy is an important part of TCM, and it is a summary of the working people's long-term experience of fighting against diseases. It is rich in content, wide in scope and long in history, and has made great achievements through unremitting efforts and exploration by doctors of all generations. TCM non-medication therapy has great advantages in prevention before disease and prevention of exacerbation, embodying the traditional academic thoughts of preventive treatment of disease, prevention over treatment, health preservation and health recuperation. After thousands of years of bumpy development, TCM non-medication therapy has fully demonstrated its tenacious vitality and strong advantages: first, its curative effect is reliable, rapid and remarkable; second, it has a wide range of indications and can be used for treatment, prevention and health preservation of hundreds of diseases in various clinical departments; third, it has a high safety. Because of the self-protection function of skin and mucosal barrier and the use of natural medicinals, the external treatment has little or no toxic and side effects; fourth, it reduces the pain of taking drugs orally.

What are non-medication therapies for health preservation?

By applying effective health-preserving techniques, non-medication therapies have the effects of keeping fit and beautification, calming the mind and improving intelligence, preventing and eliminating diseases, and prolonging life.

There are many kinds of non-medication therapies, such as acupuncture and moxibustion, tuina, massage, qigong, daoyin, cupping, stone needle therapy, fire therapy, fumigation and steaming therapy, medicinal bath therapy, wax therapy, and acupoint application therapy.

What are the contraindications of non-medication therapy for health preservation?

People with one of the following circumstances are not suitable for non-medication therapy for health preservation: with emotional impatience when the seven emotions (joy, anger, worry, thought, sorrow, fright and fear) are excessive; with fluctuating disease conditions, with high fever, being delirious, with the tendency to have complications, with disease deterioration, and serious and critical illness; being over-hungry, over-full and drunk; in pregnancy and menstruation; during thunder and lightning, storms, and scorching sun exposure; being exposed to air pollution, humid and noisy environment; with exhausted or extremely weak body; with mental disorder, or being unable to control behaviors; before and after sex.

What are the selection principles of non-medication therapy for health preservation?

Among the numerous techniques, we should make choices according to the type of the individual's constitution, the strength of the body, occupation, age, gender, hobbies, etc. As for preventing diseases, besides considering the above factors, we should also distinguish the attributes of syndromes and the characteristics of diseases, and apply techniques based on individuals, syndrome differentiation and disease differentiation.

Section 2
Massage and Daoyin

What are the basic massage techniques?

The basic massage techniques include clapping, percussing, stroking, rubbing, finger-pressing, finger-kneading, palm-kneading, finger-pinching, palm-twisting, palm-chopping, pushing, grasping and shaking.

What are the massage and daoyin exercises?

There are various massage and daoyin exercises, commonly used ones include Laozi Massage Exercise, Tianzhu Massage Exercise, Eighteen Exercises of Qigong Massage, Yancheng Daoyin Exercise, Mawangdui Daoyin Exercise, Wuqinxi, Baduanjin, Taijiquan, Frog-like Qi-circulating Exercise, Guangdu Daoyin Exercise, Turtle-like Qi-circulating Exercise, Goose-like Qi-circulating Exercise, Dragon-like Qi-circulating Exercise, etc.

Section 3
Health Qigong

What is qigong?

Qigong is an important part of TCM health preservation. It is a health care method for practitioners to exert their inner potential by adjusting their body, mind and respiration, so as to strengthen their constitution, eliminate diseases and prolong their lives.

What are the essentials of qigong practice?

The essentials of qigong practice are relaxation, quietness, unity of spirit and qi, combination of movement and quietness, and relaxed upper body with energetic lower body. The practice should be based on syndrome differentiation, combination of practice and preservation, and practice step by step.

What are the basic methods of qigong practice?

There are many schools of qigong, and they can be divided into three major categories: static exercise, dynamic exercise and dynamic-static exercise. The basic methods of exercise can be summarized as body adjustment (posture), heart adjustment (mind) and breath adjustment (respiration).

How to adjust the body?

Body adjustment refers to adjusting body posture and relaxing the body to start practice with correct movements. No matter what kind of practices, postures are always the ones to be emphasized. The correct posture is both vigorous and relaxed. "Tendons and bones should be bent, muscles should be relaxed, each part of the body should be connected, and flexibility should be integrated in it." In this way, the circulation of qi and blood will be unobstructed, creating conditions for smooth heart and breath adjustment.

How to adjust the mind?

Mind adjusting means one's thinking, emotions, consciousness and thoughts are required to gradually enter an empty and quiet state through training, so as to achieve the goal of leading qi with the mind, uniting spirit and qi, and mobilizing the potential of the body.

How to adjust the breath?

Breath adjustment refers to the adjustment and exercise of respiration. Adjusting respiration can not only directly harmonize qi and blood and exercise internal organs, but also accumulate internal qi and promote its circulation. Breath adjustment should be uniform, slow, thin, long and natural. To sum up, there are natural breath method, abdominal breath method, shutdown-closed breath method, big breath method, wind breath method, heel-up breath method, fetal breath method, rest breath method and reading breath method.

What are the common qigong exercises?

Commonly used qigong exercises include Relaxation Exercise, Standing Exercise, Internal Preservation Exercise, Zhoutian (large cirde of vital energy) Exercise, Sleeping Exercise, Mind-qi Exercise, Fame Exercise, Yijin Xisui Sutra, Hunyuan Muscle-tendon Strengthening Exercise, Liuzijue, etc.

Section 4
Commonly Used Techniques for Health Preservation

What is stone needle therapy?

Stone needle therapy is a kind of TCM-featured treatment, which uses stone tools to scrape and wipe specific parts of skin repeatedly, so as to relieve superficies and eliminate pathogenic factors, clear heat and remove toxicity, promote blood circulation to remove blood stasis, and relieve rigidity of muscles and activating collaterals.

What are the instruments for stone needle therapy?

Shuowen Jiezi: "Bian means to stab the diseases with stones." The stone used for treating diseases is called stone needle or needle instrument, which is the earliest medical device of mankind. At present, the commonly used needle instruments are divided into massage needle instrument, warm compress needle instrument, cutting and stabbing needle instrument and cupping needle instrument according to their effects and functions on the human body.

What are the indications of stone needle therapy?

The indications of stone needle therapy include: soft tissue injuries, such as acute and chronic lumbar sprain, muscle strain, and fat pad injury of the knee joint; orthopedic and traumatic diseases, such as cervical spondylosis, sciatica caused by lumbar disc herniation or lumbar spinal stenosis, degenerative osteoarthritis, and tennis elbow; rheumatic diseases, such as rheumatic arthritis and rheumatoid arthritis, scapulohumeral periarthritis, and synovitis of knee joint; peripheral neuropathy, such as peripheral facial paralysis, facial spasm, peripheral neuritis, and muscle atrophy caused by chronic neurological diseases; cardiovascular diseases, such as myocardial ischemia and arrhythmias; various functional disorders, such as chronic fatigue, insomnia and neurasthenia; beautification and weight loss.

What are the contraindications and precautions of stone needle therapy?

Contraindications: Patients with bleeding tendencies, such as thrombocytopenia, leukemia, and severe anemia; critically ill patients with acute infectious diseases and severe heart diseases; patients with skin injuries, inflammation, ulcers or initially recovered sores; patients that are over-full or over-hungry, and with fear of stone needle therapy.

Notes: Tapping manipulation is not applicable to the head; tapping and vibration manipulations should not be used near the heart; the abdomen of pregnant women should not be treated by stone needle; the cooling method on the elderly and the weak should be applied with caution; for the elderly and the weak and fragile parts of the human body, mild manipulation should be given; when using warming method, skin scalds caused by high temperature should be avoided.

What is fire therapy?

Fire therapy, a TCM-featured treatment, applies traditional Chinese medicinals with different effects on acupoints and affected parts on the body surface. Taking advantage of the heat and air convection of alcohol combustion, it stimulates meridians and collaterals, and promotes the transdermal absorption of traditional Chinese medicinals, and thus plays a role in harmonizing yin and yang, warming and dredging meridians, and promoting qi and blood circulation.

What are the indications of fire therapy?

The indications of fire therapy include: acute and chronic pain caused by wind-cold-damp bi; local pain and numbness caused by cervical and lumbar diseases; joint pain caused by osteoarthropathy; various pains caused by muscle strain and soft tissue injuries; dysmenorrhea and irregular menstruation in women caused by cold congelation of meridians; insomnia and dreaminess, cold limbs and nocturia caused by yang deficiency; abdominal pain, loose stool and constipation caused by deficient cold of spleen and kidney.

What are the contraindications and precautions of fire therapy?

Contraindications: Pregnant women; patients with severe diseases, such as malignant tumor, poorly controlled hypertension, renal failure, and bleeding tendency; drunk, emotionally unstable or mentally ill patients; patients with infectious skin diseases or skin injuries.

Notes: It is not suitable to apply fire therapy to a hungry patient, and it is advisable to apply it one hour after meals; metal ornaments should be removed before fire therapy to prevent burns; after fire therapy, patients should keep warm, avoid wind and cold, and refrain from eating raw and cold food.

What is fumigation and steaming therapy?

Fumigation and steaming therapy, a TCM-featured treatment, fumigates different parts of human body with the medicinal steam produced by decocting traditional Chinese medicinals with different effects to reach the diseased area directly through the skin and orifices, and discharges the dampness and turbidity out of the body through the opening and closing of pores, It has functions of eliminating dampness and removing toxicity, regulating yin and yang, warming meridians and removing obstruction in collaterals.

What are the indications of fumigation and steaming therapy?

The indications of fumigation and steaming therapy include: abnormal lipid metabolism; myofiberalgia syndrome; swelling, pain and limited movement of joints; lumbar muscle strain, soft tissue contusion, fasciitis and tendinitis; sleep disorder, mild anxiety and depression; obesity and subhealth status.

What are the contraindications and precautions of fumigation and steaming therapy?

Contraindications: Patients with serious diseases, such as malignant tumor, poorly controlled blood pressure, renal failure, and bleeding tendenc; patients with infectious skin diseases or skin injuries; women during pregnancy and menstruation.

Notes: The fumigation time of the elderly and those with weak constitutions should not be too long, and they need to be accompanied by their families; patients should keep warm, avoid wind and cold, and refrain from eating raw and cold food.

What is medicinal bath therapy?

Traditional Chinese medicinal bath therapy, a kind of TCM-featured treatment, can treat diseases and preserve health by combining different medicinals according to different diseases based on TCM syndrome differentiation, taking advantage of the stimulation by water temperature on the skin, meridians and acupoints, and transdermal absorption of medicinals.

What are the indications of medicinal bath therapy?

The indications of medicinal bath therapy include: joint and muscle pain, myositis, and dermatomyositis caused by wind-cold-damp bi; insomnia caused by various reasons; hyperlipidemia; diabetic foot; Sjögren syndrome; scleroderma, psoriasis, and eczema.

What are the contraindications and precautions of medicinal bath therapy?

Contraindications: Hypertension, hypotension, cardiac insufficiency; patients with large skin wounds; women during pregnancy and menstruation; patients with a history of severe allergy.

Notes: It is not advisable to apply medicinal bath therapy to a hungry patient, and it is advisable to apply it one hour after meals; water should be properly supplemented before, during and after the therapy; after medicinal bath therapy, patients should avoid wind and cold, and refrain from eating raw and cold food; the bathing time should not be too long. Weak people may experience dizziness, rapid heartbeat, nausea, soreness and weakness during bathing. Under this circumstance, the medicinal bath therapy should be terminated, and a short rest is needed.

What is wax therapy?

Wax therapy, a TCM-featured treatment, mixes traditional Chinese medicinal powder with heated medical paraffin and applies the mixture to the affected part. The soft and warm characteristics of paraffin assist traditional Chinese medicinals in carrying out local stimulation and transdermal absorption. The combination of the two plays the role of warming and dredging meridians, and promoting qi and blood circulation.

What are the indications of wax therapy?

The indications of wax therapy include: local numbness and pain caused by cervical and lumbar diseases; joint stiffness and pain caused by osteoarthropathy; all kinds of stiffness and pain caused by muscle strain and soft tissue injuries; chronic pain caused by wind-cold-damp bi; dysmenorrhea and irregular menstruation in women caused by cold congelation of meridians.

What are the contraindications and precautions of wax therapy?

Contraindications: Severe diseases, such as malignant tumor, poorly controlled hypertension, renal failure, and bleeding tendency. Drunk, emotionally unstable or mentally ill patients, and patients with infectious skin diseases or skin injuries are not suitable for wax therapy.

Notes: It is not suitable to apply wax therapy on an empty or over-filled stomach; after wax therapy, patients should keep warm, avoid wind and cold, and refrain from eating raw and cold food.

What is tuina?

Tuina refers to a kind of TCM-featured treatment method, during which doctors use their own hands to manipulate on patients' body surface, injured parts, discomfort places and specific acupoints, and use various techniques such as pushing, grasping, pressing, rubbing, kneading, pinching, finger-pressing and patting, so as to dredge meridians and collaterals, promote qi and blood circulation, help with injuries and relieve pain, eliminate pathogenic factors and strengthen healthy qi, and harmonize yin and yang.

What are the indications of tuina?

The indications for tuina include: soft tissue injuries, joint and muscle pain caused by joint sprains; hyperostosis, cervical spondylosis, intervertebral disc herniation, scapulohumeral periarthritis, etc.; headache, dizziness, hypertension, gastritis, diabetes, etc.; irregular menstruation, dysmenorrhea, amenorrhea, mastitis, etc.; diarrhea and constipation caused by deficient cold of the spleen and stomach.

What are the contraindications and precautions of tuina?

Contraindications: Acute and chronic infectious diseases, skin diseases and hemorrhagic diseases; malignant tumors, severe hypertension and heart disease; initial fractures, dislocation, and severe trauma; severe osteoporosis, and cervical and lumbar spondylolysis.

Notes: After tuina, patients should avoid wind and cold, and refrain from eating raw and cold food, and patients should drink warm water to supplement the water of the body; it is not suitable to apply tuina to someone who is too full or too hungry, and it is suitable to apply it one hour after meals.